What Makes
A Woman
Very Sexy

What Makes
A Woman
Very Sexy

❦

❦ *Julia Grice* ❧

DODD, MEAD & COMPANY

NEW YORK

For Don, whose love makes me feel like the sexiest woman in the world.

No part of this book may be reproduced in any form without permission in writing from the publisher.
Published by Dodd, Mead & Company, Inc.
71 Fifth Avenue, New York, New York 10003
Manufactured in the United States of America
Designed by Suzanne Babeuf
First Edition

2   3   4   5   6   7   8   9   10

Library of Congress Cataloging-in-Publication Data
Grice, Julia.
What makes a woman very sexy.
Includes index.
1. Sex   2. Sex (Psychology)   3. Interpersonal
attraction.   I. Title.
HQ21.G6785   1988   302'.12   87-19901
ISBN 0-396-08961-5

Contents

10

Turn-ons and Turn-offs

163

11

Sexiness in Our Lives

181

Chapter Notes

209

Bibliography

219

Index

225

Acknowledgments

The names of all persons mentioned in this book have been changed and identifying material altered to protect their privacy. My special thanks go to all the men and women who gave interviews and filled out questionnaires. I would also like to thank a number of people for their help in locating subjects to interview, providing information, or providing moral support.

These include Jean and Will Haughey, Richard Penhollow, Don Van Zile II, members of the Detroit Women Writers, Elizabeth Buzzelli, Linda Bartell, Dan Platz, Joyce Hagmaier, Pat and Sandi Scafetti, Dan Haggerty, Dick Le Roy, Michael Grice, Jr., Andrew Grice, Margaret Duda, Donna Tomlinson, Jeanette McKinney, Maria Zatezalo, Virginia Stiles, editor, *Intimate Fashion News;* the Cosmetic, Toiletry and Fragrance Association, and the National Association of Hosiery Manufacturers. A special thanks to my editor, Barbara Beckman of Dodd, Mead and to Al Zuckerman of Writers House.

Introduction

I can't remember a time when I didn't know about the existence of sex appeal. When I was ten, my cousin Stephanie, nine, was wildly beautiful. She had wide, cat-green eyes, a mane of blonde hair, and a lithe body that could dance ballet and do gymnastics. Little boys flocked after her. I, in contrast, weighed 100 pudgy pounds, wore glasses and was cursed with eyes and hair of brown.

It was a hard-learned lesson—boys like some little girls better than others. Then I thought it was because of the blonde mane and green eyes. Now I know it's more than that. It's a whole, complex combination of other factors, too. The way a woman feels about herself and her body. The way she feels about men. It's also the choices she makes, the signals she sends off to others.

Can sex appeal be learned? I believe that many aspects of sexual chemistry are controlled by how we think and how we behave. We can change the signals we send out to others, once we realize what those signals are. We can learn to behave in certain ways—use sexiness techniques, if you want to call them that.

I researched sex appeal extensively, drawing on interviews and questionnaires, and also my own personal experiences. Who has it and who doesn't? Is it a matter of body chemistry? Does a woman have to be pencil-slim in order to be considered sexy? Does she have to like men? What is the most provocative type of body language? How do you flirt? What clothes and hair-styles do men like best?

These questions and more are answered in this book, which is for every woman who ever looked at herself in the mirror and wondered . . . am I? Could I be? Do I dare?

1

What Is Sex Appeal? Who's Got "It"?

> *The plainest person can look beautiful, can be beautiful. It only needs the fire of sex to rise delicately to change an ugly face to a lovely one. That is really sex appeal: the communicating of a sense of beauty.*
>
> —D. H. Lawrence,
> *Assorted Articles*

That fascinating and fatal difference between men and women begins—literally—with the first look. Men take that first look every day, over and over again. Far more so than women ever dream of doing.

Men are extremely sexual. They have thoughts about sex—not a few times a day, but many times an hour. They "girl watch," appraising women sexually, noting their breasts, their bodies, their swingy walk. They assess how a woman might be in bed—and they even do this with strangers, women they may see briefly in the street or on an elevator. Men do this whether they are young or old, married or single, involved in a love affair or not. Couples have engaged in pitched battles over the man pausing to stare at a well-built girl walking down the street. One marriage I know began to fail the day the pair returned from their honeymoon: He glanced; she exploded.

Men do look at sexy women; they look at them constantly. This is a fact of life, a fact of the difference that is here to stay and cannot be wished or argued away. One man explained this difference in the sexes to me. "Women wear their hearts on their sleeve. Men tend to walk around with their hormones on their sleeve. In many cases the first impact of a woman is on the hormonal level. Something catches the eye—her hair, eyes, smile, or silhouette. Then, bam! This snaps the man's attention, and he makes the next move."

Chillingly—for those of us who don't feel completely confident of our appearance—this initial glance can be brief indeed. Studies have found that the average man makes up his mind in *seven seconds* whether he wants to know a woman better.

Sex appeal. What is it? Who's got "it"? William Bolitho said in *Camera Obscura,* "A very beautiful woman hardly ever leaves a clearcut impression of features and shape in the memory. Usually there remains only an aura, a living color."[1]

Is Bolitho right? Is sex appeal an aura, a glow that surrounds a woman? Or is it more a center-fold body type, big-
busted, small-waisted, curvy-hipped? Are there ways to enhance
sexiness? Hints or tricks that can be used to make one appear
more alluring, more seductive?

Since the days of Cleopatra women have pondered these
questions. And since the days of that long-ago temptress, *some*
women have been sexier than others. What are their secrets?
Is it something they are doing, or were they just born that way?
Can sexiness be learned and practiced, like a technique?

These questions are puzzling and frustrating for women
who want to attract a new male or to intrigue and fascinate the
one they've already got. How many of us have not had an experience something like this: Years ago, when I was a junior
at Albion College, I tried to fix up one of my sorority sisters
with a date for the Spring Formal. Kim was certainly not fat,
and I thought she was attractive, with her dark hair, scrubbed-
looking face, and shy ways. Yet when I asked my boyfriend to
find a date for her, he seemed curiously reluctant.

"What's wrong with her?" I finally asked.

"She's just not sexy," he told me.

I was annoyed. I'd thought Kim would make a perfect date
for one of Mike's fraternity brothers. "Why isn't she?" I demanded.

"I don't know."

"But—"

"She just *isn't*."

Poor Kim ended up staying home from the dance because
she didn't have a date. And I was left feeling dumbfounded and
irritated. What was sex appeal, that some people had it, and
others didn't, and men were the ones who decreed who the
lucky ones were? What were the qualities that Kim was missing?
Were these factors that only men could spot? Obviously, I hadn't
spotted them. Why was life so unfair?

Incident number two: Years later, as a member of a singles
club after my divorce, I met Bonnie. Bonnie was what some
call "big and beautiful." She must have weighed in at a hefty
220 pounds, a laughing, energetic, game-for-anything type of
woman who could play baseball, or go white-water rafting and
love it. Bonnie wanted to find a man, though, so she did some-

thing heroic. She went on a diet and shed about 100 of those pounds. She dieted herself down to a pencil-slim size 8 and waited for the phone calls.

The phone calls didn't come. It was almost tragic; Bonnie had struggled and sacrificed in order to become attractive to a male, and she still wasn't. In spite of the fact that she attended the singles club regularly, six months went by and Bonnie wasn't asked out.

"Why?" I finally demanded of several male friends, "Why isn't Bonnie getting dates?"

The answer: "She isn't sexy."

"But why isn't she? She's game for anything, she isn't fat, and she's a whole lot of fun."

"But she doesn't come on to the guys as sexy. She's more like a sister figure to them."

"A sister figure?"

"You know. Like a relative: an aunt or a sister."

Incident number three: Not long after that, I made a trek to my local Post Office and experienced one of life's odd, unexplainable episodes. I was 44 years old at the time, and I was wearing my usual writer-at-work uniform: a blouse and a pair of much-washed jeans. Over it I'd thrown a thigh-length car coat. My hair is curly, and I hadn't even bothered to run a pick through it, but just jumped in the car and dashed off.

It was about 1:30 PM. Returning to my car, I noticed that a late-model car was cruising past me; it pulled to a halt. There were three well-dressed men inside, all wearing business suits, and I surmised they had probably come from the nearby Main Street Seafood Bar and Grill, a restaurant that serves businessmen's lunches.

The driver rolled down his window. "Can you tell me how to get to Main Street?"

I couldn't help laughing a little: Main Street was one block away, and I told him so.

"Do you mean that way?" he asked, pointing and grinning at me as if it were all a joke. He was about my age, with dark hair tinged with gray—nice looking, even datable, if I had been looking for a date. The other two passengers, ordinary businessmen as far as I could tell, were silent.

"Yes, that way."

"But we can't find it."

"Well, you just turn right here at the corner," I began, and then gave up. The way he was making eyes at me, grinning—it was obvious that the request for directions was merely a ploy. Suddenly unease flooded me and I began to move away. Were these men trying to pick me up? Surely they wouldn't drag me into their car right in the heart of downtown Rochester at just past noon—me, 44 years old, dressed in scruffy car coat and jeans.

"Sorry," I mumbled, backing further away.

The driver's eyes and expression were intent on me, as if he was trying to communicate with me without words. Then, to my astonishment, the man reached out both hands through the opened car window, extending them to me with an air of naked pleading, palms up in entreaty. His eyes actually *begged* me. In front of two witnesses who were staying out of the matter, this man was begging to meet me!

Perhaps I should have been more adventuresome, but I wasn't. I hurried off, and as I did so I could feel the man's eyes focused on the center of my back, reproaching me. Later, driving home, I was still astonished. Those pleading eyes, those extended hands, palms up, begging. What exactly had happened? Surely those three men in nice suits could not have been planning to rape me. Not in front of the Post Office, with dozens of pedestrians scurrying past.

No, the explanation was simpler than that. Something about me or my looks or my jeans had drawn the driver's eye, sparked some hormonal reaction in him. He just wanted to meet me. He'd been hoping against hope that somehow . . . some way . . . he could make a connection with me.

What factor about me had drawn his attention? Had I looked like some other woman he knew? Was it. . . ? Could it be that he had found me sexy?

Sex appeal. A survey of 102,000 *Ladies Home Journal* readers revealed that of the women who view themselves as "traditional," 46.4 percent consider themselves sexy. Of those who feel they are "new women," 64.3 percent think they are sexy.[2]

Every woman has been forced to deal with her sexiness in one way or another for most of her life—being judged because of it, approached because of it, using it or not using it, enjoying it or not enjoying it, being complimented, whistled at, double-taked, ogled, stared at.

Cindy, one of the women I interviewed for this book, works in an automotive plant where she literally cannot walk from one end of the plant to the other without being noticed. There are whistles, teasing, comments. She has to avoid going to certain work areas because the attention she'll receive there will be overwhelming. When she filled out my questionnaire, she checked almost every item, from "men often flirt with me," to "I feared rape from a man I worked with."

What is this quality that Kim lacked, that Bonnie dieted in vain for, that drew a stranger to approach me on the street, that causes Cindy's life at the Ford plant to be a constant series of whistles and catcalls? What is sex appeal? Who's got it and who hasn't?

Men and Women Rate Sex Appeal Differently

Most people, when I asked them to define sex appeal, looked startled for a minute, as if I'd asked them something very hard. Some hemmed and hawed, and some avoided the issue altogether. Apparently it isn't easy to define something so nebulous, so based on personal preferences, a quality that, as one male writer pointed out, acts like a Rorschach test, providing clues to the personality of the one who does the defining as well.

Generally, men and women differ in the definitions they give. Voluptuous Jayne Mansfield once gave a masterfully pragmatic one: "It's just knowing what to do and then doing it with a lot of naiveté. Well, I shall be more specific. If a girl has curviness, exciting lips, and a certain breathlessness, it helps. And it won't do a bit of harm if she has a kittenish, soft, cuddly quality."[3]

Said Jeanne Duran, a former WJR (Detroit) radio personality now in her 70s, "I would say, generally speaking, if a woman establishes immediately that she *is* a woman, and that he is a man—whether it's a potentially eligible male, or just the gas station attendant—there will be a spark. And when a man feels that recognition coming from a woman, be he Robert Redford or Woody Allen, *that* woman has sex appeal."

Women tended to be far more pragmatic in defining sex appeal. The two most common elements in the answers women gave were "good grooming," and "the degree to which a woman is attractive to the opposite sex."

"It's all in the presentation," one woman I talked to declared. "It's when I look good, when I have lost the weight," said another. Other women added people-oriented qualities like "having a good sense of humor" and "being friendly." It was almost as if having sex appeal could somehow be put in the same category as being a good job applicant with certain specific, salable qualities.

Some women consider magazine-cover models as a standard for sexuality, by which other women must be judged. When my agent was selling this book, we approached several publishers. One young woman editor, evidently believing that the author of a book on sex appeal should be no slouch herself, demanded of my agent, "Is she sexy?"

"I'd say she certainly is," he responded.

"Is she sexy enough to go on the cover of *Cosmo*?"

"Why," my agent replied cautiously, "If she did, it would be too intimidating to all of her women readers."

I laughed about this later, but there was an underlying feeling of anger, too. Surely there is more to sex appeal than looking good for a magazine cover, especially for a magazine that *women* buy.

When I talked to the men, though, they were far less focused on the physical than I would have suspected. True, there were some who wanted to talk about legs and breasts. But those were far outnumbered by the men who wanted to discuss inner qualities that project sexiness—an aura, if you will. Over and over these men emphasized "inner glow" qualities in the woman, most of them having to do with sexual self-confidence. To these men, a sexy woman projects an aura. She "radiates femininity," "radiates a glow or a spark," "thinks she's sexy," and "loves life."

This whole idea of the *aura* surrounding some sexy women is fascinating. "Won't you come into the garden? I would like my roses to see you," wrote Richard B. Sheridan, in a charming tribute to this rare quality in women.[4] And in a far less poetic description, one of my male interviewees described a woman as "reeking of sex."

If anyone "reeked of sex" it was the late Marilyn Monroe. Michael Chekhov, nephew of the playwright, once said to Marilyn, "I understand your problem with your studio now, Marilyn. You are a young woman who gives off sex vibrations, no matter what you are thinking or doing."[5]

Marion Wagner, who met Marilyn when both were modeling bathing suits, said of her, "Marilyn was the most spectacular girl I ever met, not particularly beautiful, but she radiated a special dynamism. . . ."[6]

However, there is another important element to sex appeal. Over and over, in different ways, men talked about confidence. The way a woman holds herself, stands, sits, walks, speaks. Apparently confidence is so vital to sex appeal that without it a woman is—well, ordinary. And with it she doesn't even have to be gorgeous.

"A woman has to be in touch with her own personality," one man told me. "Some women have a glow, a spark, a feeling of self-worth. When a woman has low self-esteem and she shows it through her body language, it's a complete turn-off. If someone feels good about herself, then it's tremendously appealing."

"Some women breathe sex, and all it takes is one look to see it," pointed out one 26-year-old attorney. "You can see that physically they'd make a nice partner. But there's more to intercourse and love than just a good body. She has to be turned on a bit mentally. In an intimate situation, if she can encourage her partner not to be inhibited, it makes for a perfect sex partner."

A glow. Confidence. Men pick up on vibes like these right away. "Some women definitely do conform to my instincts, that know I'm right when I feel they'd be good in bed. There's a way to tell, a certain look, confirmed in the way they reveal themselves through their eyes," said an auto executive. "How? I just know that their eyes have that all-knowing look of 'I've been there, I'm looking for more.' "

The men I talked to also focused on the way a sexy woman relates to *them*. They added such factors to the definition as, "she indicates sexual availability," "she knows how to focus on the male," and "she makes a man think about her sexually." Over and over men told me that sexy women like men and relate to them well. Only lastly did many men mention physical appearance, and even then I had to prod to get them to be specific about what type of looks turned them on.

"To me," said a 35-year-old teacher, "Sex appeal is attractiveness based on sexuality. It is a hard-to-define quality in a woman that somehow promises sexual fulfillment for her partner as well as satisfaction for herself. It's a type of female 'come on' that indicates she is both available and willing to engage in sexual relations. Sex appeal involves the way a woman carries herself. . .it is far more of an attitude than an actual physical characteristic."

One nice, shy man wanted sexiness in a woman to be accessible to him. "In chemistry there are certain molecules," he told me. "One floats around—kazot! It sticks. Some aspects of women I resonate with. The way their hair is done, the smile, are very powerful attractants. When I get to know someone better, my definition of a sexy women broadens a lot. Brigitte Bardot (I guess that portrays my age) has been pushed by Hollywood as sexy, and that almost turns me off. That whole Hollywood thing is completely finished as it is, with no room for other people. I just don't picture room for another person."

A few men also mentioned another aspect of sexiness—a subtly implied, erotic danger. Rock star Tina Turner was mentioned several times as epitomizing "dangerous" sex. Cybill Shepherd has this quality, and Peter Bogdanovitch talked about it to *McCall's*. "What Cybill's always had—and what makes her popular in *Moonlighting*—is that sexual threat implicit in what she does, an innuendo. The men she plays opposite are in definite danger of being destroyed if they're not careful. That quality is harder to find than you think. Ava Gardner had it, and Lana Turner. It's not a compliment or an insult; it's a rare quality. I haven't been able to find it in any other person."[7]

Tony Scott, who directed Kelly McGillis in *Top Gun,* talks about her qualities, calling her "a striking and extremely sexual actress. It's not just purely physical because the real strength of Kelly's sexuality comes from inside, not outside. It's what's happening inside her head. It's a brooding sexuality. . . ."[8]

So here we have two different viewpoints on sexiness—the women who say that sex appeal focuses on what you do to get a man, and to what extent you are able to do it; and the men, who say that sex appeal is an attitude, an aura of confidence, a way of showing men that you are sexually available.

Women who read this book, therefore, are going to be focused on the how-to aspects. What do you do to be sexy? What actions can you take? Is there a one-two-three secret? A plan? Of course, this book will be chock full of how-tos and hints gleaned from research, and from talking to sexy women and men. But, according to the men, sex appeal is more than doing. It is also being. It comes from the inside. It glows outward like a light, drawing men to its shimmer.

I've learned from my research that sex appeal generates in many ways. It's both physical and mental. It comes from scent chemistry, from body types, from the way women interact with men, the ways they move and smile and flirt. Sexiness involves messages sent and received, either consciously or unconsciously, and it's also the way we think. To a great extent, sexiness comes from the mind.

That is good news, for what it means is this: **If sexiness is even partially in the mind, then we all have access to it.** Any woman can add to her allure, be more charismatic, more appealing. And what the men have told me bears this out. Plain women can be sexy, said the men I interviewed. Women of 50 can be sexy. Women who are 10 to 20 pounds overweight can be sexy. All it takes is that certain something, that sexual aura which we are about to study in greater detail.

Myths about Sex Appeal

When I started writing this book, I interviewed and distributed questionnaires to more than 70 men. The response was gratifying. Most were eager to talk; indeed, each man considered himself somewhat of an expert on sex appeal. After all, hadn't he been woman-watching most of his life? Actually, it was men who grabbed onto the whole idea of sexiness with the greater enthusiasm. Men who filled out questionnaires were eager to pass the survey along to others. My questionnaire became the prime topic of conversation at a Detroit Edison power pool, a

Fortune 500 company, an auto dealership, a writers group, and a telecommunications office. At one company, my questionnaire was actually sent around as a memo (presumably to spice up an otherwise dull day). And the men who responded ranged from students and engineers to salesmen and lawyers, and in age from 20 to 60.

I talked with dozens of people informally, and surveyed several dozen women writers. However, I also knew that I wanted to interview a number of ordinary women who were considered sexy by men. There was a slight problem, though: As I'd already learned, men and women do differ considerably in what they consider sexy. How could a woman accurately select another women who *men* might consider appealing? I solved this problem by asking men to recommend women to me to be interviewed. The woman had to be over 20, and could not be a wife or current girlfriend (I specified that to avoid favoritism or the feeling that one had to recommend his wife).

The 60 women I talked to provided a real eye-opener, for they did not meet my preconceived expectations at all. I thought I would be interviewing sexpots: curvy beauties with a certain wet-lipped arrogance, who were mostly in their 20s, wore plunging necklines, were physically stunning, and oozed sex.

I got a surprise. The one quality all the women seemed to have in common was warmth. The women I talked to—and, as I said before, they were all recommended to me by men who thought they were a good example of a sexy woman—ranged in age from 23 to 51. Perhaps because most of the men who recommended them were over 30, the women's ages tended to be 30 and above, too. Although all were attractive, there wasn't one magazine-cover beauty in the lot. They did not all have model-like figures; in fact, many were pleasantly curvy, and one told me she never appeared in a bathing suit or shorts unless she had to. One of the women, a warm blonde with a delightfully husky voice, had had polio as a girl, has one calf slightly smaller than the other, and walks with a limp.

Yet here are some of the things that the men said about these women: "She's a stone fox." (That was Marla, 36, a slender, fragile-looking strawberry blonde with a sweet, shy way about her.)

"There is something about her—she is the receptionist at

work, and when I first saw her I just laughed, she is so much like a Playboy bunny." (That was Renee, 24, who wears her lush mane of dark-blonde hair down past her shoulders and has a nice, solid, size 10 figure.)

"When you look at her you just know she'd be good in bed, that she'd throw herself totally into the act of making love." (That was said about Gwen, who is 40, petite, with dark curly hair and an hour-glass figure that she worries is too fat.)

"She is definitely sexy. She looks so innocent; I think that is her appeal, that she is innocent." (Dwanna, 29, is slim and black, with large, alert brown eyes and a shy, appealing poise.)

Just as I had certain preconceptions before talking to these sexy women, most of us do subscribe to some myths about what sex appeal is. For example:

- You have to be young to be sexy
- You have to be beautiful
- You must be pencil-slim
- Sex appeal is primarily physical looks
- There is only one standard for being sexy, and if a woman doesn't meet it—she isn't
- Men judge women the same way women judge women
- You have to look like a model
- Men want Playboy bunnies and Penthouse pets
- Wearing a lot of make-up will enhance sex appeal

And so forth. But the truth is that all of the above are just that—myths—and the reality is far different, or is that they are only partially true. Being sexier is within the reach of most women if they will realize one very important axiom: *Being sexy is thinking sexy. Thinking sexy will cause you to act sexier and to project sexuality to men.* In this book, I'm going to cover all the many facets of sexiness. The chemistry of sex appeal. Our bodies, and what makes them sexy. Our body *language,* all the subtle signals we give off to attract men. How to flirt. Certain "enhancement" factors that add to sex appeal. Using our minds to project a powerful sexual aura. Sex appeal in our daily lives. Choices, signals, turn-ons, and turn-offs.

You Don't Have to be 20 to be Sexy

First let's examine several of those sex appeal myths in greater detail. For instance, what about the myth that you have to be young to be sexy? Women "of a certain age" (let's say 40 to 50) are becoming increasingly visible on evening television—and they aren't playing grandmothers, either, but rather femme fatale roles. Even cosmetics companies like Germaine Monteil are using gorgeous models who are about 50, like Tish Hooker, to promote their products.

And there may be a very good reason that women in this age group are growing more acceptable as sexy. This could be simple population demographics. The Bureau of the Census reports that by the year 2000 the median age in this country will be 36.3. In fact, by 1990, the over-55-year-olds will out-number the under-35-year-olds.[9]

Mediamark Research Inc. estimated that 52 percent of the U.S. population is women, and that over 60 percent of these women are over 35. About 44 percent of all American women are over age 45![10]

Interestingly, the cosmetics industry, while vying hard for this big segment of market, does this by appealing to women's inner senses of themselves. Therefore they use illustrations of younger women or of "ravishing" 50 year olds such as Joan Collins. According to the Cadwell Davis Partners, another research firm, this might have something to do with women's age perceptions. Most adults who have reached their middle years feel 5 to 15 years younger than they really are: At 50, most people feel 35. "Many stay in their 30s almost forever in a special psychological way. . . ."[11]

This fact—that women feel younger than they really are—is a plus, sexiness-wise. To my mind, a woman who feels as if she is still in her 30s has a better chance of being confident, which will make her sexier!

Many women do worry that after they pass a "certain age," their attractiveness will evaporate, leaving them with nothing but wrinkles and memories. I can remember being 37 and having that worry myself; that I only had a few good, sexy years left. Is this a legitimate worry? How much *is* sex appeal related to age? This was an interesting question that I felt deserved looking into, so I decided to ask it, both verbally, and in the questionnaire I distributed to 73 men.

To this statement, *"Sex appeal has nothing to do with age. A woman of 50 can be as sexy as a 20 year old,"* half of the men who filled out the survey said, "sometimes," and the remainder responded either "usually" or "nearly always." In other words, most men believe a woman of 50 can be sexy. Only *one man* said "never."

"A 50-year-old woman," one man wrote, "can have 30 years more experience being sexy than a 20 year old."

Author Sidney Sheldon has said, "A body in good shape is good in bed, so even a woman of 50 or 60 can be very sexy if she's also in good shape. I think women are more sexy as they get older. Experience helps in bed."[12]

A 1984 *Penthouse* survey showed that 55 percent of the respondents said a woman's age didn't matter, and of the rest, 19 percent wanted younger women, 16 percent wanted women their own age, and 11 percent were attracted to older women.[13]

But women over 50 certainly don't get a break in the sex appeal department. As Sidney Sheldon intimated, in order to be considered sexy, they have to have exactly what all the younger women must—confidence, sensuality, and certain bodily appeals. Men emphasized to me over and over that a woman over 50 can't transmit a mother image, and "she has to have the things I consider sexy."

"Let's take Joan Collins as an example," said one 49-year-old salesman I talked to. "I saw her on TV last night. . . . God. . . . Smoothness of the facial skin is important, less wrinkles. Older women who have no wrinkles can look better than some younger women who do."

One writer in his mid-30s spoke for many men when he said he doesn't go for the very young woman. The name of the ubiquitous Joan Collins came up yet again: "To me, age is somewhat important. A truly sexy woman must be mature, somewhat worldly—no doe-eyed, innocent farmer's daughter for me. My specifications exclude most women under the age of 25. Also, many women seem to hit their peak at a later age. Consider Joan Collins, Linda Evans, Jane Fonda, and Catherine Deneuve. All of these women are over 40 and still extremely sexy. Each of them exudes sensuality, intelligence, sophistication, and self-confidence."

"My ideas about all this have changed enormously with my age (mid-40s)," said another man. "The 19, 20 year olds can be very attractive, but by my tastes today they are unfinished, they haven't paid their dues, learned any lessons. Older women have more to bring to a relationship. They aren't as new or unblemished on a physical level, but they have more attributes as people."

Physical Beauty and Sex Appeal Do Not Necessarily Always Go Together

Another common myth about sexiness is that you have to be beautiful. In the land of Madison Avenue the model who sells us perfume, makeup, and diet aids is always extravagantly, physically beautiful. Her air-brushed, perfect face shows no sign of pores, wrinkles, hairs, or shininess, and in some cases she has actually had some of her back teeth removed in order to achieve the proper, hollow-cheeked look.

In the ad she is also portrayed as sexy. Sexy and beautiful, these are the two partners, and women have bought the message that one can't exist without the other.

Of course, we know that often the two *do* go hand in hand—and when this happens we often get what is known as a sex symbol or sex goddess, such as Marilyn Monroe, Raquel Welch, and others.

But does sex appeal have to be paired with beauty? Not necessarily, according to the men I talked to. In fact, in answer to the statement, *"Even a physically plain woman can be sexy,"* two-thirds of the men answered "sometimes," and the remainder said a plain woman could be considered sexy "nearly always" or "usually." None of the men said that a plain woman could *never* be appealing!

For those of us who weren't born with a face like Christie Brinkley, the news is encouraging, especially in view of the fact that some of the men I interviewed told me that they would shy away from a woman they considered "too attractive."

Brent, a financial planner of 44, told me emphatically that

for him there is no connection between physical beauty and sex appeal. "Other than the extremes," he pointed out, "such as extremely fat. Generally speaking, I have an 'attractiveness range.' That is, a certain range of physical looks appeal to me, and if a woman falls within that range she'll be attractive to me. If I see an extremely attractive woman, it's a turn-off to me, because I'd figure I didn't have a prayer and wouldn't try, there's nowhere to go with it."

Physical beauty is definitely a factor, another man pointed out, but it is an *entry-level factor,* "important in terms of the first contact but it doesn't have sustaining power. Much more important is the ability to enjoy, to be enthusiastic. . . ."

It's all a matter of what messages a woman sends out. "Certainly a plain woman might be considered sexy if she communicates the right sexual messages," remarked another 30-year-old man. "I've known some very average-looking women who were able to come across as sexuality incarnate. It seems to be a matter of how they view themselves. Sexy women are confident and self-assured. Whether attractive or not, they seem to believe and feel that they are desirable. They are somehow able to communicate this sense of self-esteem to the male, who in turn comes to find them alluring."

Allure, inner and outer, is going to become even more important as the current man-crunch continues. A recent Yale–Harvard study showed that never-married middle-class white career women have discouraging chances of marrying once they hit 30. Still single by age 30, their chances are only 20 percent of marrying, and if they pass age 35, their chances plummet to only 5 percent.

This study scared a lot of women, who had been brought up to believe they could have it all: a wonderful, satisfying job and marriage and a family. They established careers, and now that they are ready, most of the men have been written out of the script. Potential mates are either married or looking for younger women.

One female writer speculated that the answer to the man shortage would be a renewed emphasis on coquetry, the "return of the vamp." In other words, a return to sex appeal. In the early days of the women's movement, we boycotted make-up and seductive clothes because we were tired of being seen as sex objects. Now, many women want to be sexy again, but with a different aim. Not only do they want to be sexy for a man, but they relish being sexy for themselves, too. Being sexy feels good. It feels strong and powerful.

This book will tell you how to be sexy, not only in your body but also in your mind, and not only for men, but for yourself.

Axioms of Sex Appeal

1. Men are extremely sexual and judge women on the basis of even a seven-second appraisal. As one man put it, "Women wear their hearts on their sleeves, but men tend to walk around with their hormones on their sleeves."

2. Men and women define sex appeal differently. Women think of sex appeal in pragmatic terms—that is, what they would have to do to be sexy. But men often focus on inner qualities that transmit sexiness—"inner glow" qualities that project a sexy aura.

3. Confidence is so vital to sex appeal that it supersedes other qualities. If a woman has sexual confidence, she doesn't have to be gorgeous, and if she lacks confidence, even beauty may not help her.

4. Many men believe that there is such a thing as an "aura" of sex appeal that some women project; some women give off strong sexual vibrations.

5. Men also focus on the way a sexy woman relates to them, how available she is to them, how well she focuses on them and makes them think about her in a sexual way.

6. And, there is also a subtle element of erotic danger in sex appeal, as embodied by stars like Cybill Shepherd and Tina Turner.

7. Many of us subscribe to certain myths about sex appeal—for instance, that to be sexy you must be young or beautiful or pencil-slim, or look like a model. These beliefs may be true some of the time, but not always, as the men I interviewed told me over and over.

8. Debunking myth number one: You don't have to be twenty to be sexy. To the statement, *"Sex appeal has nothing to do with*

age. A woman of 50 can be as sexy as a 20 year old," the majority of men who answered my questionnaire agreed, stating that this could be true at least sometimes. However, women over 50 musn't transmit a mother image, and they "have to have the things I consider sexy."

9. Debunking myth number two: Physical beauty and sex appeal do not necessarily always go together. Hollywood has sold us the bill of goods that sexy and beautiful are always partners, but the men I interviewed said over and over that a plain woman can sometimes be very sexy indeed.

10. The recent man-crunch has caused a resurgence in women of the desire to be seductive—but it is a new, healthier kind of sex appeal because women want to be sexy not only for men but for themselves as well.

2

The Chemistry of Sex Appeal

We may unconsciously send and receive sexual olfactory sexual messages.

—James Hassett,
Psychology Today.

Occasionally circumstances force us to be aware of the subliminal scents emitted by those around us. Once I attended a popular Egyptian exhibit at the Detroit Institute of Arts. It was mid-summer, and the temperature outdoors was at least 96 broiling, humid degrees. Those crowded into the museum, dressed in light, summer-weight clothing, were perspiring. Not only that, we were crushed together in a tightly packed line—and the humid air was apparently facilitating my sense of smell.

To my astonishment, I found that I could smell almost every person against whom the line moved me. All smelled different. One woman smelled of sweet musk and perfume and sweat. A man behind me smelled oddly peppery. Someone had had a drink before arriving at the museum, and the faint scent of bourbon mixed with a light layer of skin perspiration. Someone else had a stronger odor, more salty, mixed with after-shave. Another lady had been drinking tea. I found myself wondering what *I* smelled like to those against whom I was bumped.

Human beings *can* tell each other apart by smells alone. Fascinating and true, tests have proven this. One group of scientists was startled to discover that blindfolded subjects could distinguish each other solely by sniffing the palms of their hands. And in California, college students were given a dirty T-shirt test. For a day they sacrificed any artificial scents and left off any soap, perfume, or deodorant, and wore a special clean, identical T-shirt.

The next day each student was asked to sniff three shirts—his or her own, a strange male's, and a strange female's. Incredibly, about 75 percent of the students were able to pick out their own shirt from the others![1]

Some deaf—blind people have been able to recognize others by scent. And who among us has not stood in a crowd on a hot summer day, as I did, and catalogued the people who pressed close to us by their smells?

Scientists tell us, however, that much of our reaction to body odors may be on an unconscious level. Society has programmed most of us to push certain odors to the backs of our minds—not to "smell" them anymore. For instance, studies show that 3 and 4 year olds actually find the scent of feces and sweat pleasant, but that by the time they are five, toilet training and society's demands have overwhelmed the child's instincts.

The child is also programmed to repress other odors, such as the sexual smells emitted by his parents. One 3 year old was found to show quite strong reactions to the bedroom smells that were present after his parents had been making love. But these reactions disappeared by the time the boy was six.

However, according to psychologist C. D. Daly, subliminal awareness of such human body ordors is still there, but it is now being experienced on an unconscious level. [2]

Repressions like these can make for some interesting situations. For instance, one merchant filled two sale tables with identical sets of nylon stockings—except that one set was lightly scented. The scented stockings quickly sold out. But when customers were later asked why those stockings appealed more than the plain ones, they mentioned qualities such as texture, weave, and color. No one even noticed the true difference: scent. [3]

Janet L. Hopson wrote a whole book on the sexual aspects of smells: *Scent Signals, the Silent Language of Sex.* One of the main premises of her book is that we collect smell data on another person within the first few minutes of a new encounter. According to her, there are certain "sexual surrogate" odors such as the waft of cologne or soap that are socially permissable for us to notice. The rest we don't know that we are noticing at all. But we still notice them, and Hopson calls these potent human sex signals, *sexones.* [4]

In humans, and despite the efforts of the cosmetics industry to mask smells, there are certain body areas that produce odors. In women these are the armpit, the skin around the vagina, folds around the clitoris, the cleavage of the breasts, and the folds under the breasts. Scent glands are also found in the aurolea surrounding the nipple, in the face, hands, and feet.

Researchers say even a woman's breath can change its odor with the phases of her menstrual cycle.

Natural body scents can be heady stuff. A French historian describes a sixteenth-century ball where the Duke of Anjou accidentally wiped his face with the discarded chemise of a young noble lady, and "from that moment on, he conceived the most violent passion for her."[5] And it is probaby no accident that Victorian women often carried their handkerchiefs in their bodice, close to their bosoms.

One man I interviewed for this book told of breaking up with a girlfriend and begging her for an article of her clothing—her panties—to keep under his pillow so that he could rekindle her presence whenever he wished. And who among us has not, at one time or another, gone to the closet to take out an article of our lover's clothing, to smell its pungent, distinctive, personalized, sexy scent?

Armpit odor in other cultures has been acknowledged to be sexy, not offensive. For instance, in Greece and other Balkan countries, the men carry handkerchiefs under their arms during vigorous folk dances and then offer these pungent hankies to women to attract them as dance partners.

What does all of this mean in the arena of sex appeal? Smells are erotic and are perceived on an unconscious level. Personal odors—the kind that many women have been brought up to feel aren't quite nice—can act directly on a man's brain to heighten arousal, but at a level below awareness. If a woman wants to be sexy, she must recognize that her natural body odors may be powerful unconscious stimulants to men.

"It's funny," one man told me, "but there is something about the odor of a woman that turns me on, a certain odor that is very familiar in some women. I don't know what it is. I only know that I can be dancing with someone, and we'll both be perspiring a little, and suddenly I'll smell her. It'll be sweet and musky and so *familiar* that I'm instantly drawn to her. And this can happen even when the woman herself isn't that attractive to me in other ways. And it can happen over and over with the same woman, if I happen to dance with her more than once. Smells sure are potent."

Hopson tells the story of a Victorian man who was sitting on a streetcar bench, between his lover and a strange woman.

He smelled perspiration, and thinking it belonged to the stranger, was offended. But when the other woman rose to leave, the smell remained, and the man discovered the musky odor was coming from his lover. Suddenly he found the scent sweet, not unpleasant at all.[6]

Said one man of his girlfriend, "She smells right. I can't describe it any better than that. I love her smells, and that is the trouble I have had with some other women I've met. They just don't smell right to me."

Years ago I attended a dance feeling very depressed. I was newly divorced, a too-quick romance had collapsed, and I felt very lost and alone. I was standing uncertainly at the edge of the dance floor, watching the milling singles who apparently all were having a better time than I was, when a short, bearded, blond man asked me to dance.

Reluctantly I agreed. He told me that he was a sailor on a Great Lakes freighter—and I told him I was a writer. It was clear we had little in common, yet for some reason I told him I had just broken up a relationship. "You poor thing," he said. As we continued to dance, something began to happen. I smelled him—the clean, soapy, faintly tobacco-smelling odor of a healthy, virile man.

As the music continued I began to experience odd feelings of familiarity and ease. His natural odors had so many associations for me of past men I had known: my father who had held me on his lap, a beloved grandfather, a husband, a lover. The dance lasted only a few minutes, yet when we parted I felt calmed, released, comforted.

Incidents like these point out some of the fascinating aspects of "odor homogamy," the fact that men and women are drawn to each other because of their odor configuration, a comfortable feeling when the sum of a person's skin, hair, food, and workplace smells spell out, well, home. Perhaps in a more primitive world, such odor homogamy had a real purpose—to guide humans into mating with those who were similar.

But our bodies have evolved from the animal, and animals do rely on odors to transmit powerful sex messages. Human beings might suppress their responses to sex odors, but animals certainly don't. In fact, sex in the barnyard wouldn't even occur without the strong influence of smells.

A case in point. There is a substance called "boar taint," emitted by the male pig's sweat glands, salivary glands, and a gland in his foreskin. It is so powerfully sexual that it literally controls copulation between the male and the female. When the female sniffs the "boar taint," she automatically stiffens into a rigid position for mating. Farmers call this behavior the "immobilization reflex." If they can smell the boar, 90 percent of sows will stand rigid and wait for sex, *even if they can't see the boar.*

Some enterprising farmer capitalized on this aspect of pig love, and invented an aerosol can filled with "boar taint," which is used to make the sow stand still for artificial insemination!

Other clever farmers ready their goat herds for mating by rubbing a billy goat from another farm with a rag, then stuffing the cloth into a tin can. Curious female goats nuzzle "Billy in the can," and usually come into heat soon after.

With horses, it's the scent from the female that gets the sex cycle going. Ranchers who are trying to collect semen from studs to use in artificial insemination sometimes spread the urine or vaginal secretion from estrous females on "teaser animals" to get the males in the mood.

Primates are a step upward from barnyard animals, and much closer to man's own evolutionary ancestry, a fact that has not been lost on scientists who have been trying to study chimps and monkeys in search for clues to human behavior. Female rhesus monkeys have several ways of attracting mates. Anyone who has ever seen these animals in a zoo knows what I am talking about. The female rhesus—literally—waves a red flag at males, for during her fertile days her rump grows bright red and hot.

"This flood of hormones affects her mood as well," says Janet Hopson, author of *Scent Signals.* "And sexiness oozes from her posture, her expressions—and maybe her scent glands."[7]

One scientist, R. P. Michael, suspected that indeed, a vaginal odor signal might be partly responsible for primate sex appeal. He decided to study this. Doing research on monkey couples, he discovered the female secretes a substance he calls "copulins." Just as the name implies, the substance, containing five fatty acids, proved to be a powerful stimulant to male ardor; it is a veritable monkey aphrodisiac.

In fact, Michael learned that he could make a synthetic mixture of these chemicals that was nearly as powerful as the natural one, and could even be rubbed onto a second female without ovaries, to invoke male passions.[8]

Which brings us to an interesting question: Do human females also secrete a version of "copulins" that attracts males on an unconscious level?

Michael studied that, too. And he decided to go straight to the heart of the matter by studying tampons that had been used by human women—in fact, he analyzed 635 tampons used by 47 women throughout their menstrual cycles. What he and his team learned was fascinating. Nearly all of the tampons (97.5 percent) showed at least some trace of the volatile fatty acids dubbed "copulins." However, 14 of the 47 women produced *much more* of these so-called copulins. In fact, they secreted so much of the substance that the scientists called them "producers."[9]

Do sexy women produce more copulins than other women do? Is this one of the secrets of their extraordinary appeal? It is a question that will occupy scientists for many years to come. But scientist Michael did state that anxiety over vaginal odors may be "quite misplaced."

One nineteenth-century French physican—and fancier of women—came up with a system to describe that delicate, elusive *parfum de la femme*. Professor A. Galopin said that a woman's very personal scent all depends on her hair color. Blondes emit the scent of ambergris; while chestnut-haired women give off a violet scent; and brunettes the odor of ebony wood and musk. The French doctor claimed that meat eaters smell stronger than vegetarians (an observation echoed by others), and that the skin of older women smells like "dry rose leaves or decaying linden blossoms."

And of course there is the memorable quote from novelist Tom Robbins, "O vagina! Your salty incense, your mushroom moon musk, your deep waves of clam honey breaking against the cold steel of civilization. . . ."[10]

The sexiest women know, because men have told them,

that musky female odors are a strong attractant. Not dirty odors—men say that uncleanliness is a real turn-off—but sexy ones. When I questioned men for my survey, half of the men said they found natural female body odors either "extremely appealing" or "fairly appealing." About one-third said these odors were "not important," and less than one-quarter said that natural odors were a "turn-off." (And some who said these smells were a turn-off were referring to after-tennis funkiness.)

Part of sex appeal, men pointed out to me over and over, is when a woman really likes her body and feels relaxed inhabiting it. Body-liking and odor perception may go hand in hand. If a woman thinks that her natural scents are repugnant, she's going to feel less good about herself, and this means she'll carry herself in a less confident manner.

The media has convinced most women that their bodies smell bad, because they want to sell us millions of dollars' worth of products. Remember the big advertising campaign in the 50s to get all of us feeling bad about "B.O.," so that we would buy deodorants. Now there are sprays and douches and advertising to frighten women into feeling that they might have vaginal odor.

But sexy women need to feel good about their bodies. How can we feel alluring when we're worrying that we might offend? We can't. Women who feel less than confident about their body scents (and I use that word deliberately, because it implies something more pleasant than the words *smell* or *odor*), need to talk bluntly with some men on this subject. What they would learn might be very surprising.

"I heard that Frenchwomen put their fingers in their pussy, then touch their fingers to their neck, etc., using it just like perfume. It *is* a perfume. I think that the natural female body smell is very erotic," bluntly stated one of the men I interviewed for this book.

If you feel uneasy about your own body scents and tastes, perform a little experiment on yourself. Wait until some private moment when you are naked, relaxed, and alone. Then sample yourself as a man might do if he were making love to you. Rub your fingers in your vagina, then smell the fluids, sample their aroma. Taste them. Rub your fingers along the sides of your groin, near your pubic hair, where scent glands proliferate. Rub under your armpits, and in the folds between and underneath your breasts. Sniff your skin, sampling its delicate scent. *Are these smells and tastes really repugnant to you? Aren't they actually rather sexy, in a funky, musky sort of way? And, in your heart of hearts, don't you find the same odors in your lover to be equally intriguing? So why shouldn't he enjoy them in you?*

Appealing odors.   Men really do respond to natural female odors; in fact, these powerful scents turn many men on. Are you worried about bad smells when you're out dancing? Here is what one man told me. "I have almost never smelled bad body odor on the dance floor. I go to dances about three times weekly. And you know how hot it gets with all those people doing fast rock dances. It's good, clean sweat and that doesn't have a bad odor at all. What does turn me on is when I dance with a woman and I can smell *her.* Maybe it'll be the scent of her hair, or just the soft smell of her skin, or the soap she's used. Maybe it's her femaleness. I don't know what. It just turns me on."

A woman of 32 told me about an encounter she had with a former boyfriend, with whom she had just broken up. "We went out for a drink, and Jack started reminiscing about all the times we'd been together in bed. I'll admit there was still a lot of physical chemistry between us and that kind of talk did turn me on. Afterwards, he walked me out to my car. I got in the car, the door was still open, and he stood there with this look on his face. He told me that he could smell me . . . *me.*

"I told him he was crazy, he was standing three feet away, he couldn't possibly smell that. But he insisted that he did, that it was just as strong as could be, and it was driving him sexually crazy. He started coming on strong to me right in the parking lot. I could scarcely believe it, that my female smells could be affecting him that strongly, but I could tell he meant what he said."

Brigitte Bardot, the international sex symbol of the 60s, literally reeked of sex. Dr. Richard Gordon frequently visited sets where Bardot was acting, and he remarked that her distinctive bouquet was caused by overactive endocrine glands.

He commented that he had observed the "same sweet muski-ness only a very few times in his medical career, and always on very highly sexed women."[11]

So if we want to be sexy, let's be proud of our clean natural smells, not ashamed. Encourages one man: "I think a woman should maintain personal hygiene, but not to mask certain odors that are a part of her. If she feels good about herself using an artificial deodorant, fine. But she shouldn't be afraid of her own natural body odors, if she has no medical problems—just let them shine through."

Axioms of Sex Appeal

1. Our sense of smell is much stronger and more detailed than we think. Human beings can tell each other apart by odors alone, and tests on blindfolded subjects have proven this.

2. However, because society has programmed us to think certain smells are "unacceptable," most of our reactions to body odors may be on an unconscious level.

3. We collect smell data on another person within a few minutes of the first meeting. Some smells, like those of perfume and after-shave, we permit ourselves to recognize, but others we don't know we are noticing at all.

4. There are certain body areas in women that do produce sexy odors—the armpit, the skin around the vagina, folds around the clitoris, cleavage of the breasts, folds under the breasts, aurolea surrounding the nipple, as well as the face, hands, feet, even the breath.

5. There is an interesting factor called "odor homogamy," when men and women are drawn to each other because of their odor configuration, which is a comfortable sum of a person's skin, hair, food, and workplace odors.

6. Animals rely on odors to transmit powerful sex messages, and, after all, *we* are descended from the animals.

7. Scientists suspected that a vaginal odor signal might be partly responsible for sex appeal in the female rhesus monkey and dis-covered a substance called "copulins."

8. Human women were studied for the presence of "copulins" by examining menstrual tampons, and it was learned that some women (the sexier ones?) secreted much more of these so-called copulins—so many that the scientists called them "producers."

9. The media has convinced women that their bodies smell bad and that they should feel shame about themselves. But the truth is that natural female body odors may be an important part of sex attraction; to wash them all away might be a mistake.

10. Men generally *like* natural female odors and many men respond powerfully to them.

3

A Sexy Body

*Her cheeks like apples which the sun
hath rudded,
Her lips like cherries charming men
to bite,
Her breast like to a bowl of cream
uncrudded,
Her paps like lilies budded,
Her snowy neck like to a marble
tower;
And all her body like a palace
fair. . . .*

—Edmund Spenser,
Epithalamion

Standards in female beauty change from century to century, decade to decade. Witness the great, *zaftig* models painted by Reubens and Renoir with all their flowing pinknesses of flesh. Today those women would be considered obese. But in some cultures, because most people led hard, debilitating lives, it was considered sexy if a woman had a lot of poundage, because that meant she was too wealthy to have to work.

The great beauties of the Edwardian era were all "big girls" weighing over 150 pounds. The famous beauty, Lillian Russell, had a 42" bosom, and a 27" waist that was achieved by super-tight corseting. Raved the *New York World* about this stellar creature, "All the undulations of the prima donna's figure modeled graciously in ripples that were so many sonnets of motions."

Lillian's rival, Anna Held, was equally solid. Although she was under five feet tall, her measurements (tightly corseted) were a hefty 36-20-36.

Harriet Hubbard Ayer said, "The beautiful arm should be round, white, and plump" and the phrase "she has no thighs," meant that somehow a woman was sexually thin and inadequate. The chorus women on the cover of the *Police Gazette* were by our standards fat, as were women on the burlesque stage, actresses, chorus girls, and the women pictured on cigarette cards. Even the early Ziegfeld Follies girls, in all their glory, had firm round legs that were by no stretch of the imagination slim. [1]

Dieting didn't start until about 1895. Actress Fanny Davenport went on a diet in 1889, and Lillian Russell in 1896 began to watch what she ate when unkind reviewers began comparing her to a "white elephant."

Suddenly, in the 1920s, the flapper appeared on the scene—narrow where women had always been wide, binding her breasts to appear flat. Suddenly full bosoms were no longer fashionable, and it was the thin-bodied look that counted.

The Hollywood starlet of the 50s was taller and more slender, her measurements approximately 35-25-35, but since exercising hadn't yet come into vogue, she tended to be somewhat flabby. One photo showing six shorts-clad starlets standing in a row, reveals that they all had slim legs, but their flesh did not have the kind of tight, aerobic-exercised definition that we all take for granted today.

Aerobics, popularized by people like Jane Fonda, has wrought vast changes in the way women in the 80s view their bodies. Cher goes on television to tout an exercise spa, showing ripples in the muscles of her back. Now it's fashionable to be not only slim, but tight, and women bodybuilders, once considered grotesque, are increasingly being recognized as attractive.

"The new bold beauty is round; she's not scrawny," says Francesco Scavullo, the renowned photographer. "Her body looks healthy and strong enough so that you could wrestle and roll with her."[2]

Male Criteria for Women's Bodies

The first woman a young boy is in love with is, of course, his mother. Later in life many men are unconsciously drawn to women whose bodies resemble, in some loose way, their mothers'. We all know that mothers—especially of the nonaerobic 40s and 50s—were built like ordinary women, probably tending to be slightly plumper and less-exercised than women of today.

One man I interviewed for this book told me that the type of woman he is sexually drawn to is "curvaceous, not slender, tending to a hint of plumpness, with a rounded derriere, melon-like breasts, and a look that says 'I enjoy making love.' " Later, for some reason, our discussion turned to mothers, and he told me that his mother also had a voluptuous, large-breasted figure, and was, as he put it, "sexually liberal and open." The description of the woman he wanted matched that of his mother.

It comes as no surprise to women to learn that men put physical features first when looking for a purely sexual relationship. This may, in fact, be a survival quality for the human race, since a nubile, sexy young woman would probably be a healthier one, better able to produce more children.

Studies have shown that blue-collar men tend to be drawn to a woman with a heavier figure. Extroverted men like women with fuller breasts, and men of European or Arab background also like the fuller-bodied woman. Some primitive tribes are turned on by pendulous breasts, which probably represent age, revered in those tribes. Other African tribesmen love women with extremely rounded, protruding buttocks, and sometimes young men used to select brides by lining up all the available girls in a row, and selecting the one whose buttocks stuck out the farthest!

One group of researchers questioned college students on how important 53 qualities were to them in choosing either a one-night stand or a more meaningful, long-term relationship.

When they wanted a long-term commitment, both men and women put "inner beauty" first—qualities like honesty, fidelity, and sensitivity. But when it came to the purely sexual, the men veered sharply. The top ten qualities they wanted were nearly all physical, having to do with a woman's body. In order of choice, these were: the woman's figure, her sexuality, her attractiveness, facial features, buttocks, weight, legs, breath, skin, and breasts.[3]

As more than one man pointed out to me, "The first time you see a woman, all you notice is the physical, that's all there is to see. The rest of it comes later, after you've noticed her that first time. The first time she opens her mouth to speak, that's the real, acid test."

Some Men are Partialists

We've all heard of men who say they are "breast men," "ass men," "leg men," and so forth. The technical term for someone with this kind of preference is partialist, and sexual partialism is extremely common among men of all types.

According to William A. Rossi, an authority on the foot and shoe who has researched these kinds of preferences, "Most men are partialists. They have their own personal preferences for women who are tall or short, thin or plump, blonde, redhead or brunette . . . high or low-slung buttocks, etc. A man will say, 'I'm partial to blondes with small feet.' Another says, 'I like women with large bosoms and small waists.' Still another says, 'I'm a leg man.' Each is a partialist."[4]

"Woman as a whole is a desirable object," says clothing historian James Laver. "But man cannot take all of her in at once. He is therefore compelled to concentrate on one particular part of the human body."[5]

Partialism is so common that we see it evidenced all around us. I'll never forget a first date I had with one man who told me that he was drawn to women with attractive legs. They had to be full and firm, with nice, tight calves, and as he was telling me this, he actually reached down under the table to feel my calves!

Another man told me he has been cruising singles clubs for months, looking for this woman: "She should be tallish, thin, with dark hair and high cheekbones and pretty eyes. Some people might call them squinty but they are the type of eyes I like; and she has to have a certain cute look to her."

And here is what one college professor would order up if he could: "Physically she is a dark-haired brunette of French-Italian extraction, 5'3" to 5'5", and normal weight."

"A blue-eyed blonde, curvy, that would be my preference," said another man.

Even celebrity men are specific in the body types they prefer, according to an interesting little book I picked up, entitled, *What Makes A Woman G.I.B. (Good In Bed)*, by Wendy Leigh. Says Wilt Chamberlain: "I really prefer dark-haired girls with dark eyes, olive skin, nice legs, and nice strong buttocks which have a little protrusion. The breasts can be any size as long as they are firm and not altogether sagging."[6]

Omar Sharif: "I don't particularly like slim women too much myself. . . ."[7]

French superstar Charles Aznavour: "I like boyish women, unformed, not exactly finished. . . . For my Pygmalian ego, I like to have a teenager in bed."[8]

And actor Oliver Reed: "My ladies should be voluptuous. I like large arses."[9]

Jimmy Connors wants someone soft: "I am pretty picky about ladies. Part of my pickiness is that I like them not too skinny nor too fat—I like a little bit to hold onto. I like ladies with very smooth, very soft skin I can nestle up to and cuddle with. If I could choose the best woman in bed for me, I would like one lady: very soft, very smooth, very gentle, very cuddly, pinchable, squeezable. . . ."[10]

(By the way, that phrase "a little bit to hold onto," is a telling, very typical male expression, used to express a desire for a slightly fuller figure than most women think a man wants.)

Partialism, then, may sound unfair to some women—if a man prefers large breasts, and they happen to wear B cups, they may feel slighted. But partialism actually is a benefit for most of us, because what it means is that a wide variety of women can be found sexually attractive, at least by some men. Tall women, short women, muscular women, blondes, brunettes, large-breasted and small, each of us owns a segment of devotees and admirers. This segment may be large or small, but it does exist. As one 28-year-old woman who has modeled "big and beautiful" clothing and wears about a size 20, explained to me, "Yes, I find men, all the men I want. But I need to meet *more men* in order to do so."

But what happens when a man becomes *too* turned on by one part of the body? Then this is no longer partialism, but becomes a sexual fetish, passing into the annals of sexual abberation. Unlike partialists, a fetishist adores the body part more than he does the woman herself. If he is a hair fetishist, it is hair he grows passionate over, to the point of obsession. Forget the woman, he loves her hair. Fetishists frequently and literally *make love* to their favorite part of the body, or even items of clothing.

Nineteenth-century author George du Maurier was a noted foot fetishist, and he wrote some flowery odes to the beauty of female feet. For instance, he describes one woman's feet as "Astonishingly beautiful . . . such as one only sees in pictures and statues—a true inspiration of shape and color, all made up of delicate lengths and subtly modulated curves and noble straightnesses and happy little dimpled arrangements in innocent pink and white."[11]

Du Maurier was more than just "partial" to dimpled feet— he idolized them, worshiped them as the most sexual part of the whole anatomy. Even greater foot fetishists were men in old China in their worship of the bound feet of their women. These tiny, folded-over feet were euphemistically called "Golden Lotuses," and were sexually much desired. The bound, fore-shortened foot actually created a deep crease where the toes were bent over. This crease the enamored man likened to a second vagina and even used in that manner in lovemaking. Men literally made love to the "Golden Lotus," never mind that the poor woman whose feet were treated in that manner endured years of pain as a young girl and could barely totter as an adult.

Fortunately, however, today most women don't have to contend with the peccadillos of the fetishist. Indeed, there are many men who don't focus on specific preferences at all. In a recent singles ad page in the *Detroit News*, of 59 men who had placed ads, only 26, less than half, stated they had a body-type preference for their dates. Some of the men I interviewed also revealed that they had no preference.

"It's the total package I'm interested in," one man told me. And another added, "It's so varied. "If she is well kept, takes care of herself, has a positive image in her body language and holds her head up . . . that's what I really want."

Penthouse and Playboy Women

One prevalent myth about sexiness is that men deeply prefer women who look like centerfold models for the "flesh" maga-zines, and to the extent that a woman does *not* look like these bare-all models, she is *not* sexy.

One 32-year-old woman told me about a fight she had with her boyfriend over this very topic. "Kent showed me this huge stack of *Penthouse* magazines that he'd been hoarding. I leafed through them and saw all these gynecological pictures that were just displays of genitalia—period. I couldn't understand how my boyfriend could get so excited over what was basically hair surrounding a hole, if you want to be frank about it.

"He kept trying to explain to me how men get aroused by quick stimuli like that, and I got mad at him. I don't look like those women in *Penthouse* and I never have. I figure if he could desire one of them, how could he desire me? We had this huge fight about it. He kept trying to explain that it had nothing to do with me, and I couldn't stop being mad about it."

What woman does not exist who has not thumbed through one of the "flesh" magazines, only to be puzzled and angered? If men really want those women, what hope is there for the rest of us, who don't look like centerfold models now, and never did, even when we were 20? Is this type of spread-legged, reveal-all, heavy-lidded, blatant type of sexuality what men really want?

I decided to ask this question of the men I interviewed, and almost universally they agreed that the "pets" and "play-mates" are fantasy, not real life. (However, according to sex experts, men *are* turned on by the sight of female genitalia—this is definite fact.)

One male writer told me: *"Playboy, Penthouse,* and other magazines like this present fantasies which I feel are primarily masturbatory in nature. These publications give their readers the "perfect" woman—beautifully shaped, unblemished, smiling beguilingly or gazing out from lust-narrowed eyes. Of course, real women are simply not this perfect. I believe that most men realize that these magazines are dishing out fantasy, but what does it matter if fantasies ignore reality? The models are essentially gorgeous plastic nymphs without personalities. They are works of art positioned, lit, and airbrushed by a photographer. These women remind me of those rubber, lifelike, inflatable dolls that sailors once used while away on long voyages. They serve a purpose, but God help the man who believes they're representative of real females."

Many men remarked that the *Penthouse* women only exist on the printed page, and aren't alive and breathing. "If I were to meet a live woman who doesn't look half as good, but she's there and alive, she can be more sexy," one said. "Personality plays such an important role."

Agreed another man: "The feelings that the *Penthouse* women cause me to have are very, very different from the feelings I'd have for someone I was attracted to. The reality of a true erotic relationship is not what I'd get from pictures. There's no person there. As soon as a real person is involved, it's a different thing."

Indeed, if a woman who looked like one of these super-voluptuous models were to walk into a room, many of the men present would shy away from her, for fear of rejection. One of the men I interviewed confessed to me that he is one of these. He says he can't approach a woman who is too attractive. A few days later, I happened to meet him with his girlfriend, and she bore out his preferences. She was of average looks, middling-plump, and wore no make-up.

"Someone extremely beautiful scares me," said another man, a computer programmer. "To me that would be over-challenging. Someone like a model would have sex appeal in an unattainable way. The *Playboy* type of sexiness is not realistic. If I see a woman on the street, and she's superfoxy, I'm not impelled toward her at all. . . . I like more the Sally Fields type."

There are some things we can learn from *Penthouse*—I'll point these out in Chapter 8. However, women who worry about the *Penthouse* and *Playboy* standards, fearing they can't measure up, are only eroding away at bits and pieces of their own sexiness. *Many* women are sexy, all different kinds of women, and in all different physical and mental ways. That is one of the beauties of human diversity.

A mathemetician and philospher once was musing on just what constituted the perfect woman. He started by looking at the wide number of physical features that must be considered in declaring a woman "beautiful." There are, for example, the nose, the ears, the hair, lips, shape of the head, breasts, buttocks, waistline, and so forth. Mosciewitzky postulated that there might be twelve required features, with ten degrees of perfection for each. He concluded that it would take 10 to the 13th power woman, or one in a hundred million million, to find one perfect woman—that is, many thousand times more women than are alive now, or who have ever lived on Earth throughout its history!

Part of Sex Appeal is the Contrast between the Male and Female

One way of describing a physically attractive female is almost deceptively simple—she is "not male." This is the theory advanced by British sex researcher H. J. Eysenck, who explains, "This might seem fatuous, but what it really means is that physical attraction is based on the differences between the sexes. The points of maximum difference between men's and women's bodies are most attractive and arousing, and the more exaggerated are those differences, within reason, the more sexually attractive they will be."[12]

Sexpots—famous sex goddesses—owe part of their allure to the fact that they do maximize the difference between male and female. The "average" woman, for example, might have a waist that is only 8 to 10 inches smaller than her bustline. But along comes Raquel Welch, with measurements that are notably different. Estimates of Raquel's figure range from 37-22-35 to 40-24-36. That's a voluptuous 16 inches of difference between bust and waist! And Marilyn Monroe is said to have measured a curvy 35-22-35. Again, an exaggerated 13 inches.

Models for the flesh magazines tend to have larger breasts than the average woman. Evelyn Treacher, the first cover girl for *Penthouse,* measured 36-23-36 and Stephanie McLean, the magazine's first "Pet of the Year," was an hour-glass 40-25-36.

On the other hand, print models, who really must appeal to women, need to have a figure that tends to the other direction, *minimizing* the difference between the sexes. To have a chance with a New York modeling agency, an applicant needs to have a narrow figure measuring approximately 33-22-34. As Peg Bracken once quipped, "This wild, emaciated look appeals to some women, though not to many men, who are seldom seen pinning up a *Vogue* illustration in a machine shop."[13]

Other aspects besides measurements point out the vital, exciting difference between male and female. Soft, smooth skin without hair, so unlike a man's thicker, rougher, bearded skin. Fuller lips, narrower eyebrows, softer complexion, relative hairlessness of arms and legs which women further emphasize by shaving or depilating. (One reason men hate hairy armpits and legs is because they too much resemble the male norm.)

Large breasts are sexual because they are so softly, curvily different from the flat male chest. A female's walk evokes desire because her pelvis is wider, causing her hips to swing in an alluring, nonmale manner. *Nonmale,* then, is the key, and to the extent that a woman can capitalize on her features that make her different from men, she is sexy.

In Body Types, for Every Turn-on, There is a Turn-off

When I quizzed men on what body types they preferred, I expected to learn that one type or another would be considered more desirable, while another type would be less alluring. What I learned was exciting and far different. In some cases, what turns one man on, turns another man off.

For instance, when I asked men about their preferences in height, the answers were varied. About one-fifth of the men said they were turned on by a tall woman, but nearly one-fifth were turned off.

"I really go for a tall woman," said one. "Five-seven is a minimum, I like them real tall, and I would even be drawn to a woman who is six feet in height."

One man told me he was going to look for only tall women, as a result of a marriage that folded in part because the height difference destroyed the pleasure of lovemaking. He was 6'2". She was 5 feet tall. "There were fourteen inches difference in height between us," he explained. "And when we were in bed, I couldn't look into her eyes when we were making love. It drove me crazy. We tried all different sorts of positions and we just couldn't do it—her eyes would be about at the level of my rib cage. We just weren't compatible in height. Now one of the things I look for in a woman is her height. She has to be at least five-six or five-seven, minimum."

What about the short woman, then? She also has her devotees. As one female psychologist, a petite 5 feet in height, told me, "Men really like the short women, they really go for it, they're crazy for it. I've had them falling over me most of my life."

This woman was happily drawing the approximately 20 percent of males who are attracted to short women. In my brief study, one-fifth of the men thought a woman about 5 feet tall is a real turn on, and but an equal number, about one-fifth, were turned off.

Or let's take another type of body, the woman with a "model type" figure, pencil-slim, with the lean look of the professional model. I expected that men would overwhelmingly vote in favor of this svelte woman. After all, hasn't the media brainwashed us into expecting that a sexy woman looks something like the cover girl of *Glamour?*

Yes, two-thirds of the men responded in the two upper answers; they found a pencil-slim figure either "extremely appealing" or "fairly appealing." But nearly one-third of the men responded more negatively. Seventeen said they found the model figure "not important," and nine said they found this look a *turn-off*. A model figure a turn-off? Yes, that's what these men said.

And one-third of the men I polled said they would find a woman who is 10 or more pounds underweight a turn-off, while only four said they'd find a super-thin woman "extremely appealing."

Another example is the woman who pumps iron, and has a muscular, bodybuilder's type of figure. It bothers many men to meet a woman who can press 485 pounds and is stronger than 50 percent of the male population.

Carla Dunlop, a top female bodybuilder, told an interviewer, "I've even been called a transvestite. One time I got off the train in Manhattan, Grand Central Station. I had on jeans and a tank top, my hair was down, and as I walked along the platform a conductor who was standing there just backed away from me and started screaming. I mean he really freaked. 'What the fuck is this? You call this a woman? She's got bigger arms than me!' A couple of weeks later, though, I ran into him again, the same guy. I had on a yellow dress, totally backless, and of course I was showing even more muscle, but I was wearing make-up and the guy whistled. So you see, a lot of the response is traditional. There's no in-between. People either compliment you or they're hostile."[14]

When are muscles too many for sex appeal, as defined by the average male? I had assumed that most men would find this look undesirable. I was partly right. Yes, nearly half of the men rated the muscular look a turn-off. But the rest did not! In fact, four rated this look "extremely appealing," and 17 said that it is "fairly appealing" to them.

What all of this means is that whatever body type you have, there will be at least some men who find it a real turn-on, and more who find it moderately pleasing. Good news indeed for the woman who worries that her tall (or short, or full, or muscular) figure will turn off men.

Men Like a Fuller Figure than Many Women Believe They Do

Now we come to the matter of weight, a bug-a-boo for most women, who tend to be fat phobes, fearful that even a few excess pounds will make them undesirable. Repeated studies have shown that at least three-fourths of American women feel they are too fat, *even when they are of normal weight.* This fat-fear penetrates right down into the grade schools. I know a woman who put her 5 year old on a diet so the child could get into her designer jeans. A third grade girl took a dislike to her new teacher, because the woman was obese. Indeed, a new survey has revealed that 70 percent of fourth grade girls are concerned enough about their weight to diet![15]

Further, college women misconstrue the type of figure that men really like. One study quizzed both men and women on ideal body types, and asked them how closely they themselves matched that ideal. Repeatedly, the young women overestimated how fat they were, and said they thought the men liked a female figure far *thinner* than the curvier shape the men said they actually were drawn to![16]

Models may be the ideal for some, the fantasy for others, but the larger woman is here in America in vast numbers. The garment industry estimates that one-third of the entire female population—25 million women—wears a size 16 or larger, and according to Royal Woman, a mail order firm that caters to "big and beautiful" women, if you add those women who wear a size 14, that figure jumps by 30 million more.

Is being fuller-figured the death knell for sex appeal? Not if a woman is less than 60 pounds overweight. (Nearly all the men I surveyed, with the exception of four, said they found the woman who is 60 or more pounds overweight a turn-off. More on this later.)

But what about the woman who is slightly overweight, say,

10 to 20 pounds? One-third of the men I polled said they found a woman like this "fairly appealing" and more than a third (31) said the extra poundage "wasn't important." Only 15 said this would be a turn-off for them.

I rephrased the question, and asked men how appealing they found a woman with fuller curves, *"not overweight, but with 'something to grab onto.' She may wear a size 12 to 16 dress."* The majority of men were even more enthusiastic. Most rated this type of curvier figure as "extremely appealing," and more than half found it "fairly appealing."

One day I was strolling through a bookstore with the special man in my life, and we paused to thumb through a calendar that featured page after page of pin-ups sprawled in provocative poses, clad in little nothings that were low cut and high thighed. Don flipped through the pictures and finally pushed away the calendar, turning to me.

"These women aren't sexually attractive," he remarked. "Not to me."

"They aren't?" I asked, stunned and pleased.

"No," he said almost angrily. "They aren't, they're just too emaciated, why, they're all skin and bones. Ugh, I want something to grab onto in a woman."

I was smirking a little to myself as I left the bookstore, because I wear a size 12 dress and my figure could best be described as "curvy." Fuller than the models' in the calendar, fuller than Joan Collins', and yet men are attracted to my shape.

But what about the woman who *is* a larger size, who tips the scales at 50, 60, or more pounds beyond what the weight charts say she should? *A fat woman is a quilt for the winter,*[17] is a Punjabi proverb, and we have all seen heavy women out in public who are being treated super-attentively by a man who obviously loves and cares about them.

Women should realize that no matter what their size, there is a man who wants them. A year or so ago, I was in a greenroom in a Minneapolis TV station, publicising an earlier book, when I met a whole bevy of women who were modeling queensized clothing. They were curvy, confident, and happy, and we sat for forty minutes or so, discussing how we felt about our bodies and about ourselves.

Most of the women had finally come to terms with the fact

that they were not reed-slim and probably never were going to be. They had learned to like themselves the way they were, and this self-liking showed in the way they dressed, and the way they carried themselves. They were like bright, beautiful birds.

One 28-year-old woman, a gorgeous size 20, told me that, yes, she was able to find men—all the men she wanted—but she had to meet more people in order to do so. *Meeting more men* is the secret. Earlier I told you that most of the men I interviewed found women 60 pounds or more overweight to be a turn-off. But *four* were not turned off. Since I talked to 73 men, these four represented 5.5 percent of the total. By these ratios, if a heavier woman were to meet 100 men, even briefly, she would be likely to run into 5 who desired her type of body, and if she met 500, that number would jump to 27.

Some "big, beautiful" women are doing just that—placing themselves in a position where they will run into more men who do like their body type. Leslie, a woman I know, is about 90 pounds too heavy, a warm, outgoing, "Earth mother" type who never lacks for friends. Leslie is very active in several singles groups where she has been able to meet and talk with many men.

Bud was Leslie's choice, a man who is of normal weight, warm, loving, and even talking marriage! Says Leslie with a catch in her voice, "He told me that he doesn't care if I ever go on a diet. I don't have to lose weight for him as long as I'm healthy. He tells me that I make him laugh the way he hasn't laughed in thirty years."

There is a dating service in New York called "Plump Pals," that specializes in finding dating match-ups for heavyset women, "the bigger the better," according to owner Rita Kenny. Ninety-five percent of the men who use her service are average sized men who want to meet a heavy woman.

"These men," Kenny says, "want to meet a woman who looks and feels like a woman. There are a hundred reasons. Some men are insecure; some are looking for a mother figure. For most of them big is beautiful. Thin is out, voluptuous is in."[18]

Three years ago, Kenny's daughter, who weighs in at 350 pounds, was working at Atlantic City's Tropicana Hotel, and told her mother that European men were always asking her out and expressing interest in her. This gave Kenny the idea for her dating service.

Ed, one man who uses the service, is a research specialist from New Jersey, who is 6'1" and weighs 190 pounds. He said he joined Plump Pals because he wasn't happy with the women he had been meeting. "I knew I was attracted to heavyset women in the past. I don't care what society thinks. I just know what I'm attracted to."

On his second date, he met Barb, 5'4" and weighing 255 pounds. Immediately he was drawn to her. "I would be attracted to Barb if she was 150 pounds, 250 pounds or 350 pounds."

The moral of these stories is plain: Even a large woman needn't give up in the sex appeal department.

A Sexy Face

What makes a beautiful face? A lack of extremes, discovered one nineteenth-century photographer, Sir Francis Galton, who asked himself that very question, taking dozens of photographs and then superimposing them all on the same negative. What he got was a single, average face. Features common to most of the faces were retained, while too-long noses, eyes set too close together, blemishes and peculiarities were eliminated.

"The result," Galton said, "Is a very striking face, thoroughly ideal and artistic, and singularly beautiful."[19]

Many of the men I talked to described various parts of a woman's face that they considered exceptionally alluring, many of them mentioning the eyes. One man wanted a woman to have a certain type of wide bone structure around the eyes. And of course, wide-set eyes are one of the qualifications for a candidate to become a magazine model.

"Sex appeal in a woman is in her eyes first," said a 30-year-old accountant. "It's the sparkle that draws a man, it's the confidence, the pleasure in herself, that the eyes exude. Eyes are also a wonderfully seductive lure."

Some also mentioned the mouth, telling me about women who wore lipstick that was "red and wet," mouths that were just a bit arrogant.

"Kind of pouty, maybe full lips," one man specified. "One

of the guys at work, he's got this girlfriend, and she's pretty young but she's got a great mouth. She wears a wet-looking lipstick."

For years romance novelists have described women with a "sensuous mouth," and this mouth is usually full-cut, rosy, slightly pouting, with a prominent cleft in the upper lip, and a full lower lip. There is reason for this description. During erotic arousal, the lips become swollen and redder, so any person whose lips are fuller, more protuberant, or highly colored, will transmit heightened sexual signals.

Lipstick is a way of heightening mouth sexuality, a fact women have sensed for generations. It is no accident that in staid and sexually repressed Victorian times, it was considered very "fast" and shocking for a woman to apply color to her lips, and the only women who dared do so were actresses, mistresses, and courtesans.

A fascinating sidelight on lip coloration was revealed in Dolly Parton's biography. The nubile, eager, and irrepressible teenaged Dolly longed to wear lipstick but her father wouldn't let her. So Dolly solved the problem by painting her lips with mercurochrome. The mercurochrome hurt, but it didn't come off, and Dolly got her wish to have sexy, red lips.

Even the blush that women brush on their cheeks has sexual meaning. Blushing, says Desmond Morris, author of *Body Watching,* has also come to be linked to sex appeal, mainly because flushing is a characteristic of the sexually young and inexperienced. Today's youngsters (many of whom get experience early) tend to be more blasé, but in past years blushing was linked to flirtation and courtship. It still has connotations of sexual shyness and virginity. In fact, in ancient times, girls being auctioned off at slave markets fetched a higher price if they were blushing!

According to Morris, humans have been conditioned to respond to the round cheeks and tiny, budlike noses of babies as infantile and appealing. Grown women with this feature can elicit the same sort of doting, protective feelings in men. In other words, the shorter and more tip-tilted a nose is, the sexier it is. As Morris remarks, "A model girl or an actress who possesses an unusually small nose . . . appears not only appealing but also beautiful."[20]

Voices, too, project sexiness, and the key here is that the voice should seem not-male. Men tend to like a voice that is soft, rather than hard, and that suggests femininity, although a certain huskiness or breathiness may be appealing. "I like voices," one salesman told me. "A sweet, soft voice, not raspy like smoker's voices. You can always tell a smoker."

"But it has to be natural, not worked on," cautioned another man in listing his preference for a breathy voice.

"An interesting voice," specified another. "And how about interested?"

Women who want a sexier voice should keep it light and soft. Trish, who is in telecommunications, told me that her voice is her strong point and often men flirt with her over the phone. Several blind dates even began to fall in love with her telephone voice. "Why? I think it's because I always try to keep my voice bubbly and light and happy," Trish speculates. "My voice is clear. I speak enthusiastically, I laugh quite a bit over the phone, and I guess I try to talk as if my voice were a smile."

Facts and Myths about Breasts

Breasts are indisputably another symbol of female sexuality—one of the "differences" that spurs sex appeal. A rather amusing study was done of driver response to hitchhikers, by C. Morgan and associates at the University of Washington. These researchers planted various types of hitchhikers along the road. They learned that male drivers were more likely to stop for a female hitchhiker when her bra had been padded![21]

Breasts are sexual signals, in the same category as buttocks, believes behaviorist Desmond Morris. He theorizes that in primates, the females display their sex-signals from the rump-view, as they walk around on all fours. But a human female walks upright and when she is talking to a man, her "unique paired hemispheres," the buttocks, are concealed from view.

Therefore, says Morris, "the evolution of a pair of mimic buttocks on her chest enables her to continue to transmit the primeval sexual signal without turning her back on her companion."[22]

Another analyst has a different theory. Says therapist Lucy Freeman, author of *What Do Women Want? Self-Discovery*

Through Fantasy, "One reason large breasts are envied, by both men and women, is that in fantasy they represent the penis—a breast projects from the body, is an erogenous zone and (in lactating women) ejects a fluid. In some primitive tribes, women bind their breasts so they protrude stiffly in front, like an erect penis."[23]

But whatever the theories, no one will disagree that breasts are sex symbols, especially not women who have spent lifetimes agonizing over the fact that they feel their own are too small or too large.

As author Colette said, referring to breasts, "How do you like them? Like a pear, a lemon, a la Montgolfiere, half an apple, or a canteloupe? Go on, choose, don't be embarrassed. . . ." According to undergarment industry surveys, the majority of women in this country wear a B cup, (or half an apple.) The breakdown goes like this: 15 percent wear an A cup, 45 percent wear a B cup, 29 percent wear a C cup, 8 percent a D cup, and the remaining 3 percent, wear larger than a D cup.

But which do men prefer? Men like breasts, period, is what I learned from my survey, when I quizzed men on their preferences for breast sizes ranging from Dolly Partons (D, DD or larger), down to small breasts (A cup). In fact, a number of my respondents went right down the list, marking either "very appealing" or "fairly appealing" to *all* the breast sizes listed.

The inimitable Dolly Parton has always celebrated her large bosoms, even exaggerating them on occasion, and has been quoted as saying, "If I hadn't had them I would have had some made."[24] But how appealing were these extra-full breasts to the men in my survey? Eight of the 73 men I polled said they found "Dolly Parton" type breasts to be "extremely appealing," with 19 saying they found them "fairly appealing," and another 19 "not important." A fact that should reassure many women with a smaller bustline, about one-third of the men said they found such large bosoms a turn-off.

The most popular size of breast, however, was the full-breasted C cup. More than half the men I questioned said they found C cups "extremely appealing," and nearly all the rest found full breasts "fairly appealing." Only one of the men found C cups a turn-off.

Men who do like large-breasted women, studies have

shown, tend to be extraverted in personality—the outgoing type who date frequently, have plenty of male interests, read *Playboy,* and are independent. On the other hand, men who prefer smaller breasts tend to be more introverted and quiet, holding fundamentalist religious beliefs, sometimes being more dependent and mildly depressed.[25]

What about average-sized breasts? Women who wear a B cup can take heart. In my informal study, B cups ran a very close second to C cups, with more than a third (29) stating that they found average-sized breasts "extremely appealing," and more than half finding them "fairly appealing." None of the men found B cups a turn-off.

Women with small breasts often feel needlessly self-conscious. I once received a fan letter from a woman who had agonized over the size of her A cup breasts, until she had convinced herself that most men, when they met her, were judging her solely on the size of her bosom.

"Jewish men," she agonized, "want their women to be *zaftig.*" She talked about rejection after rejection, all based on the "fact" that she had A cups. I finally wrote back telling her that it was her *thinking* her breasts were inferior that was projecting in her body language to these men. Feeling inadequate was making her hunch her shoulders, slump, and act unconfident and unsexy.

Small breasts do have their devotees. Anthony Leonard gives them this flowery tribute in *Forum:* "It has been my observation that of the women I've known whose erotic responsiveness has been most intense, sharpest, most urgent, most highly pitched and peaked . . . that of those women who are most likely to feel sexual in an acute, sharply piercing way, most have relatively small breasts with relatively large nipples. That is, they possess more erectile tissue in ratio to fatty tissue."[26]

Most of the men who responded to my survey said they found A cup breasts either "fairly appealing," or "not important." Ten said they found small breasts "extremely appealing," while 9 said they found them a turn-off. The moral here is that it is actually a very *small* percent of the male population who find A cup breasts a turn-off—most men don't mind.

What does all this discussion of breast size mean in relation to sex appeal? If body-confidence is one of the prime factors in a woman's feeling sexy (and it is), then *no matter what a woman's size,* if she feels confident that at least some men are going to find her attractive, she has a better chance of being sexy. And that belief is absolutely true. No matter what a woman's figure type, there is somewhere a man who is crazy for it.

Sex Appeal and the Pelvis

There may be some behavioral basis for the common male preference for women with widely curved, feminine hips. Believe it or not, studies have been done on the shape of human pelvises, and how this affects sex appeal. As is well known, males tend to have a narrower, funnel-shaped pelvis, while the female pelvis is tube-shaped, and relatively broad at the bottom, causing her to have wider hips, a swingy walk, and a more awkward run.

A German physician, Dr. W. Schlegel, researched this extensively, and found that the shape of the pelvis actually varies from person to person within each sex. That is, some men have wider pelvises, and some narrower, and the same goes for women.

He discovered that behavior is correlated with pelvis shape. Men and women who have funnel-shaped (male) pelvises, tend to behave in a masculine manner, while people of both sexes with tube-shaped (or female) pelvises, tend to behave in a feminine manner. A feminine type pelvis correlates with empathy, suggestibility, and compliance!

Schlegel even studied cows, whose pelvic outlets are easier to measure than are those of human subjects. He learned that cows with narrow outlets (male-like pelvises) tended to mount other cows and generally to behave in a more masculine manner!

More interesting tidbits unearthed by Schlegel: gay males tend to have feminine-shaped pelvises. And married couples with "concordant pelvises" (both shaped the same) were much less likely to be divorced![27]

In terms of sex appeal, this may have significance. Remember, an exaggeration of femininity, of the differences between the sexes, is alluring for men. The wider the hips are, apparently, the more feminine is a woman's behavior. This may be what some men sense when they say they are drawn to a woman with "curves"—the innate femininity that curviness represents.

The Sexy Leg and Foot

Women who want to realize the full potential of their sexiness need to know that many parts of their body—not just the obvious ones, can be sexy to a man. In researching this book I came upon some fascinating sources, and none was more interesting than a book that held the unlikely title of *The Sex Life of the Foot and Shoe,* by William Rossi. Rossi, a podiatrist, is an avid and thorough researcher into the social aspects of the foot and shoe. In his book, he covered such chapter headings as "The Erotic Foot and the Sexual Shoe," and "Thank Your Foot For Sex." Humorous as these headings might be, they pinpoint the author's contention that *feet* are an erogenous zone that many Americans tend to ignore.

Here in America we have been trained to be "foot cripples," to think negatively about our feet, to view them as tired feet, smelly feet, big feet, or as an object of humor. We spend millions of dollars yearly on foot antiperspirants, and consider foot odor one step (pardon the pun) below underarm odor.

Actually, as foot experts point out, it is only shoe-wearing people who complain of "offensive" foot odors. Specifically, it is shoes that cause odors. The human foot, tightly encased in leather or plastic for 16 hours a day, produces odor when it reacts with the chemicals in the shoe. The unadorned foot, contends Rossi, is not of itself bad-smelling. Among non-shoe-wearing people there is rarely found any excessive foot perspiration (bromidrosis), and this has been confirmed by investigators in Africa, China and India.[28]

Although this knowledge is repressed in many people, the foot is actually a very sensuous, sexy area of the body. It is ripe with nerves, and is one of the lesser-known erogenous zones. The sensation of a tongue being drawn slowly between the toes is highly pleasurable for many, and there are reports of women who have been able to have orgasms from having their feet fondled.

Sexy women, as more than one man pointed out to me, have an instinctive feeling for this kind of sexuality. "Linda Ronstadt sings barefoot, and I find that incredibly sexy," a man told me once.

I attended a discussion group on a hot summer night, and found Bev, my hostess, padding around without her shoes, apparently perfectly comfortable. Two men, learning of my book, took me aside to tell me that I ought to interview Bev as a sexy woman.

"You have sexy toes," Karen's husband tells her regularly, pointing out what he considers their best features; the fact that the toes are short, with the second toe not longer than the first. "To me, my toes look perfectly ordinary; to him, they are little jewels," Karen said ruefully yet proudly.

Whether it is shape, breasts, hips, or even feet, the female body is ever mysterious and intriguing to men. It has been immortalized in poetry and song, praised for its beauty and symmetry and grace. And yet each woman is different in some way, and that is as it should be. Sexual allure is broad enough, wide enough, to encompass a variety of body configurations. If it were not, if only *one* type of female were desirable, then either all women would look alike, or the human race would have died out long ago.

Axioms of Sex Appeal

1. Styles in bodies change, and the beauties of the Victorian and Edwardian era were, in our terms, fat. It is important for women to realize this, and to know that these heavier women were considered as sexy in their day as Raquel Welch is in hers.

2. Men do put physical features first when looking for a one night stand, but tend to look for other qualities when it's a long-term relationship they want.

3. Some men are "partialists," that is, they are drawn to certain body parts above others, and consider them extremely sexy. Partialism is actually a benefit for most of us, because what it means is that a wide variety of women can be found sexually attractive, at least by some men.

4. Most women feel inferior to *Playboy* and *Penthouse* centerfolds. But men generally agree that these tantalizingly posed sexpots are fantasies, not real life. And some men admitted that, if a *Playboy* model walked into a party, they might not approach her anyway.

5. One way of describing a physically attractive female is that she is "not male." Famous sex goddesses like Marilyn Monroe and Raquel Welch have body measurements that boldly accentuate the differences between the sexes. Exaggerating femaleness is sexy. Exaggerating maleness isn't.

6. No matter what a body type is, or how alluring some males may find it, other men will find it unappealing. For every turn-on, there is a turn-off.

7. Men like a fuller figure than most women believe they do, and the majority of the men I surveyed said they find a woman with fuller curves, who is ten to twenty pounds overweight, either "fairly appealing," or "extremely appealing."

8. A woman who is 60 pounds or more overweight is rated as a turn-off by most men—but not by all. Heavier women must meet more men that the slimmer woman in order to find a possible mate.

9. One quality of a beautiful face is a lack of extremes. A small nose lends sex appeal because it appeals to the part of a man that also responds to babies, kittens, and puppies.

10. A sexy voice is one that is sweet, soft, light, non-threatening, and has a smile in it.

11. Breasts are sexual signals, and the majority of women in this country wear a B cup. The most popular breast size to men was a C cup, followed by a B cup. However, women who feel self-conscious about having small breasts may be making a mistake; only a small number of males find A cups a turn-off. Many of the men I surveyed simply liked breasts, whatever the size.

12. Women should know that criteria for women's bodies vary tremendously from male to male. There is no "one" standard for being sexy, a fact that opens up sexiness to most of us, if we choose it to be so.

4

Sexy in the Mind

*If a woman hasn't got a tiny streak
of a harlot in her, she's a dry stick as
a rule.*

—D. H. Lawrence,
Pornography and Obscenity,
This Quarter (Paris) 1929.

While interviewing men for this book, I was usually seated across a table from them with a golden opportunity for flirting. One man, 47 years old with a handsome face and prematurely silver hair, kept making it very clear to me that he thought not only that I was "very nice," but also that I should be one of the sexy women in the book. One of the questions I asked him was only half serious. It was, "If you could sit in a hot tub with three women, which three would you pick?"

He named, without hesitation, Raquel Welch and Julia Grice. Then he told me he couldn't think of any other woman to finish off the trio. Later, after the interview was over and we'd begun talking about ourselves, Jim suddenly stopped the conversation, stared at me, and said, "Take Raquel Welch out of that hot tub."

Driving home, my thoughts kept returning to this very responsive man. I knew instinctively that with just a few bits of body language, I could have had Jim half-falling in love with me. But all through the interview, I'd had the feeling that I was controlling my sexuality. Since I already had a serious relationship, I did not want Jim to come on too strongly. Yet at the same time I wanted him to like me enough to be willing to agree to distribute some of my questionnaires among his contacts at a suburban singles group.

Somehow, it had all worked: Jim was interested, but not too interested; he agreed to help me; we parted with the friendliest of feelings. What were the real dynamics of our interview? How was I controlling it?

Thinking back, I realized that several things had been happening. First, much of sex appeal is certainly unconscious behavior—over which we don't have absolute control. Yet certain thoughts were present in my mind, coloring the way I behaved. The first of those thoughts was: *This is an attractive man, this is a sexy man.* I found that I was looking at his hands and seeing them as hands that could make love. I was looking at his body and seeing it as a slim, conditioned body in good shape for sex.

The second thought running a subtle counterpoint in my mind was about myself: *I am sexy, I am very attractive, he is finding me that way and I know I look my best tonight; I really look very nice.*

Because I held the thought in my mind that he was sexy, my unconscious body language projected this thought to him. There was a synergistic effect. He felt sexy because he sensed that I thought he was sexy. Because I was thinking that *I* was sexy, I was able to project my own sensuality. These two factors—my thoughts about his sexiness and mine—were what caused him to be attracted.

Also, my body language was classic flirtacious behavior. That is, I used a great deal of eye contact, but I lowered my eyes from time to time, whenever the sexual vibes got a little too strong. I touched my hair with small, "grooming" gestures, I toyed with my drink glass, I smiled a lot, and I used some shoulder shrugging.

But how did I control all this sexiness, so that we were able to part with a friendly sexual zinginess between us, no hurt feelings, and no strong come-on on Jim's part? By the third thought in my mind, which was: *I already have a boyfriend whom I love, and I'm meeting him later tonight.*

The thoughts that a woman has in her mind—and the way she feels about herself and men—are vital in projecting sex appeal. There cannot be sex appeal without several different kinds of thoughts: One, that the woman feels attractive; two, that she finds the male attractive; and three, that there exists within her a certain innate sexuality.

When I quizzed men on their views of what a sexy woman is and how she behaves, one picture emerged startlingly clearly: Many of the qualities of sex appeal have less to do with bodily beauty than they do with *how a woman thinks.*

According to these men, a sexy woman usually looks as if she likes sex, and she talks or hints about sex at least sometimes. She is sexually less inhibited in bed (19 of the 73 men said "nearly always" and 28 said "usually.") She is comfortable with her own body and usually aware of her own sex appeal. She seems to like men as people, not just as lovers. She seldom treats men in a cold, rejecting way, and she often seems sexually drawn to the man in question. She often acts sexually available.

Ladies Home Journal, in 1982, asked 83,000 readers for their responses to a sexual questionnaire. In an interesting sidelight, the magazine separated out the responses of the 12 percent of the women who described themselves as "excellent" lovers, and who pictured their marriages as being "very sexually satisfying." *LHJ* compared these "sexiest wives" to the least sexually satisfied of the respondents, in the process learning more about what makes some women sexier.

These LHJ "sexiest wives" overwhelmingly loved sex. They saw it as a pleasure, not a chore, made love three times as often, and set aside lovemaking time with their husbands, even making dates for sex. They felt good about their bodies and only 6 percent thought their sex life would improve if they were younger or thinner or looked better. It was, the authors of the survey agreed, partly their *attitude,* their mind-set, that made these wives sexier than the other women surveyed.[1]

Of the men and women I talked to, most said the same thing over and over in different ways: It is a quality of mind that often makes women sexy. Said one man, "A sexy woman is admitting that she likes you and finds you attractive and still exhibits an air of confidence in herself. *If she sees herself as attractive, she'll project attractiveness. Even if you have two women with pretty general physical characteristics, the one who thinks she's more attractive will be more attractive.*" (Italics mine.)

Psychologists and sex therapists know that one secret of sex appeal is that many women are turned on by their own attractiveness—a healthy kind of narcissism. As one 24-year-old office worker told me, "Being sexy depends more on how you feel about the way you look than the way you actually look. *If you're accepting of your appearance and feel good, then this will come through. Other people are going to see that and think of you as attractive.*" (Again, the italics are mine.)

Claire Rayner wrote in *New Woman,* "Sexual awareness . . . is a very close relative of self-esteem in that a person who has it is conscious of her own sexuality and takes pleasure in it. Knowing yourself to be a woman, enjoying being a woman, allows other people to share your knowledge and joy. It has nothing to do with obvious sexual characteristics. *A woman who feels herself to be sexy, will be."*[2]

"Any woman can be sexy if she wants to be," one attractive man of 35 told me. "If she just lets herself let her hair down, that's really all it takes, *just her wanting to do it badly enough."*

Mind-set then is vitally important in sex appeal, turning the ordinary woman into a seductress, even when other conditions are equal.

Sexy Women Like Men

Several years ago I was having coffee with a woman friend as we gossiped about our lives and discussed the foibles of men. She was still married; I was single and looking. Suddenly Sally set down her coffee cup with a click.

"Why, Julie," she exclaimed. "You still like men, don't you?"

I stared at her, startled. This question wasn't on the subject at all—yet maybe, in another way, it was. "Yes," I admitted. "I do."

She said, "I have to confess that I don't anymore. I really think that women make much better friends. Oh, don't get me wrong, I'm not lesbian or anything like that, and I still want a man around for—you know—financial reasons and sex. But I don't think I really like them. They just aren't good friends, warm friends, in the same way that women are."

For months afterward I thought about this conversation, mulling it over in my head. Yes, I decided, I really do like men. I enjoy being with them, their humor, their protectiveness, confidence, bravado, their secret weaknesses and vulnerabilities. There is something about male companionship that you just can't get from a woman, and this holds true with very young men—16 or so—and men all the way up to their 70s. There is always a feeling of sexual appreciation. Men enjoy you as a woman, even if you are not in a relationship with them. I guess I enjoy being enjoyed as a female.

And Sally doesn't feel this? The more I thought about this, the sadder I became for my friend. If she doesn't like men, then

Sally is projecting this attitude toward them with every word she speaks, every movement of her body. Because people *know* when someone doesn't like them. They intuit it through body language, words left unspoken or emphasized in the wrong way, and facial expressions that say, "I don't trust you."

Sexy women do like men as people, most of the time, and this genuine liking of males may be one of the secrets of the deep appeal of these women. After all, men have said over and over that *they like the women who like them.* The bulk of the men I polled said they thought sexy women like men "usually" or "nearly always," while only a small minority said "sometimes."

"Sexy women like themselves," remarked a 30-year-old accountant. "And they enjoy life—they probably enjoy men, too, kind of in that order."

A tool-and-die maker added, "My experience is that sexy women like people, and generally speaking they will have lots of friends, both male and female. People who don't like people aren't sexy, it doesn't matter how good they look."

The sexy women confirmed this, most of them saying that they do like men and think that men make good friends. Most said they had male friends. In fact, many specified that they like men *better* than women. A 35-year-old teacher whose blonde good looks attract stares told me, "Men are less catty and petty than women are. When I taught high school I loved the boys, not because I had the hots for them, but because I had a better rapport with them than with the girls. Sometimes women and women don't mix, there is that competitiveness, jealousy or whatever. My mother feels the same way. I suppose I learned that from her."

Sexy women—at least the ones I surveyed—don't have debilitating feelings of anger toward men. Indeed, usually they like them. "My best friends in each period of my life have been men," says Jenny, 29. "I like men a whole lot—not better than women, or maybe I do. Women have a lot of traits I find it hard to deal with. I don't want to be negative so I'll tell you what I like best about men. They look at the whole picture more, they see someone doing something wrong and they don't say, 'Okay, what a bitch,' they say she must be having a bad day. They take the whole person into consideration, not just one act. Men are less apt to play games, more apt to say what they think."

Zsa Zsa Gabor, to whom sex appeal is as natural as breathing, has expressed similar sentiments. "I have always attracted men naturally. I like men and I like to sleep with men that I like. Obviously, I am not a cold woman; a man likes a woman who is not cold, and I think that they recognize that in me . . . some women are much more receptive to men than others because they are born to like men. They are not just sexy, they like being with men."[3]

And Joan Collins, sex appeal personified, recently told an interviewer, who asked her what made her sexy, "Maybe it's because I really like and appreciate men, and like the company of men. And I really enjoy being a woman a lot."[4]

Do you think that men make good friends? Do you enjoy being in the company of a man even if it isn't sexual? Do you consider yourself fairly free of angry or bitter feelings toward the male sex? Would you feel deprived if you were suddenly forced to spend all your time with women? If you can't answer yes to these questions, you're probably sending out negative messages to men, and diluting your sex appeal.

Sexy Women Like Their Bodies

Sexy women like their bodies more, and are pretty well satisfied with the way they look—far more so than the average woman. Nearly all the women recommended by men for my survey said that they liked their body "usually" or "nearly always." This is in striking contrast to the general population. More than half of all women don't like their bodies very well, or are actual fat-phobes, terrified that they are overweight.

Repeated studies have shown that the majority of women feel too fat—whether or not they actually are. When *Mademoiselle* quizzed its readers in a survey, the magazine learned that 79 percent of those who responded were either underweight or of normal weight, yet 65 percent of these same women believed they were too fat. *Three-quarters* of these women wanted to lose from 5 to 25 pounds. Only 6 percent were "very satisfied" with their images in a mirror, and nearly half were either not very satisfied, or not satisfied at all.[5]

Renee, 29, has "good days and bad days." On her good days, she wakes up in the morning, looks in the mirror, perceives herself as attractive, and puts on something zingy that shows off her body. She goes out into the world and is treated for what she is—an attractive woman.

"But the bad days . . . ugh, then it all changes. I wake up and I look at myself in the mirror naked and I see all the saggy places, the pouches at my stomach, and the cellulite on my thighs. I start feeling like a blimp, I feel disgusting, and that's when I go to my closet and pick out something to hide behind—something big and baggy like a tent." Wearing her dark-colored "blimp dress," Renee shuffles around for the rest of the day, hating herself, feeling fat and unattractive.

People who feel fat, *act fat*. And don't we all know what fat behavior is? It's wearing our blouses outside our pants or skirts to hide stomach bulges. It's refusing to wear shorts or tight pants, refusing to wear sleeveless blouses or anything that might reveal our "fat" body. It's walking along without much spring in our steps, knowing that if any men pass by on the street they won't be looking at us. It's feeling self-conscious when we are around men, hoping they aren't staring at us too closely. It's not wanting to undress in front of our lover, or not wanting to make love with all the lights on, but rather in pitch blackness, so he can't see the fullness of our stomach. In fact, studies have shown that 16 percent of women do have exactly these fears in making love. They are afraid the man will see their body and be repelled by it.

The sexy wives in the *LHJ* survey preferred to make love in low light, rather than in the dark—showing that they had high feelings of body esteem.[6]

But what of the woman who hates showing her nakedness to a lover? Says Dr. Sheila Jackman, codirector of the Division of Human Sexuality at Albert Einstein College of Medicine, Bronx, New York, "This attitude stems from an 'I don't like my body' problem. This is probably *the* most common reason many women believe they're too fat, too skinny, too lumpy, or have bad skin. They think that men are going to spend time studying their naked bodies. The reality is when men are enjoying sex, no one stops to count pimples or note how big breasts are. The partner is totally involved and couldn't care less."[7]

Need I say more? Women who feel fat walk around without much confidence, and their body language projects this as accurately as if they wore a sign proclaiming *"I'm Not Sexy."* Remember, confidence is half the secret of sex appeal. Men pick up confidence vibes . . . and *body* confidence is the most seductive of all.

It's a fact that most women—even actresses and professional models—focus on *some* aspect of the body that they find less than perfect. Actresses must attend "cattle calls" where hundreds of women are judged by appearance, and this tough competition makes even the most striking women insecure about their looks. If a blonde is wanted that day, and a woman is brunette, she can feel inadequate even if she is beautiful.

But even ordinary women seem to feel this touch of competition, judging each others' looks and their own with sometimes brutal harshness. This is apparently an eradicable part of femininity, at least in the 20th Century. However, the sexy women I talked to seemed more immune to this syndrome. They would tell me things like, "I'm not comfortable in a bathing suit; I don't have a teenaged body, I have a 36-year-old body, but that's worth something, too, and there have been no objections. Really I would like to look like something out of a beach movie, but I guess it's not that important because I'm not willing to do the work."

My body has things wrong with it but basically I'm happy with it, seems to be the statement most of these women made. Several didn't like their skin: one had a pigmentation problem; one couldn't get a suntan. For others it was breasts or heavy legs or "bulgies." But they spoke about these problems lightly, philosophically, assuring me that "every woman has her good days," and telling me about the many compliments men had paid them in spite of these so-called defects.

One woman I talked to is a charmer, with a cute, curvy figure, a mop of curly, dark hair, and a face that lights up when she talks. "Like my body?" she remarked thoughtfully, "I'm pretty comfortable with my body; my belly is too big and too flabby but I can deal with it. I complain about my stomach but then a man tells me he thinks it's cute, a woman should have a bit of a belly."

The truth is that men perceive sexy women as being happy

with their bodies. If you're not—if you feel miserable when you look at yourself in a mirror or when you're around attractive men—you can bet that your body language is allowing these feelings to show. A woman who can like her body pretty much *as is* has a far better chance of being considered sexy than one who dislikes her shape.

As most of the men believed, these women are also aware of their own sex appeal—they usually know they are sexy and are comfortable with that fact. This type of sexual confidence is enormously appealing to the male.

"A woman who is sexy always leads you to believe that she knows you're observing her, that she's kind of leading you on," remarked a mid-level executive for an auto company. "It's all a formulation of how they signal, how they feel about themselves, a coordination of various body parts. I always have the feeling they know they are being watched—and that they enjoy that feeling."

A male college professor agreed. "Frank body language commands an interest. Don't try to hide, don't get embarrassed over the way your body is. Sexy women look at a man when they talk to him, and aren't afraid to stick their boobs out, it doesn't bother them to have a man look at them."

Part of sexual confidence lies in not being too anxious over the men who—apparently—aren't attracted to you. A sexy woman accepts the fact that she can draw some men, and doesn't waste time yearning after the ones who aren't interested.

One thing I quickly learned as I was thrown into the singles world after having been married for 16 years, was that no matter how pretty I felt, or how many compliments I received, there were always men who didn't find me attractive. I could attend a party and have 6 or 7 men eagerly trying to meet me or take my phone number—while 100 others went about their business, which didn't include me.

And yet over and over I was to learn that some of that ignoring was deceptive. For one thing, I discovered that often men look from a distance but don't approach. Several times I had the experience of having men come up to me and say that they had been watching me for several weeks, or they had stayed away because I had been talking to someone else. Later, I began to make male friends, who told me stories of shyness and reserve. They would go to parties and observe women from afar, nervous about approaching because she "might be married" or "was too attractive" or "was already involved with a guy."

Age May Add Significantly to Sexual Confidence

Perhaps increasing age can *add* to sex appeal in some ways, rather than detract from it, as women fear. Interestingly, a number of the women recommended to me were over 35, and most of the women I talked to said they feel better about their bodies now than they did when they were younger—no matter what their age. Is it because they've had more time to receive positive feedback from men, in turn making them feel sexier than ever?

Recently, while cleaning out my basement, I happened upon a mildewed box stuffed with old high school and college yearbooks. Fascinated, I thumbed through it, turning first, of course, to the photo of myself at 18. I had gone through my high school years feeling clumsy, heavy, and just not very pretty, so it was a real surprise to see that girl who stared up at me from those old yearbook pages. She was pretty and incredibly fresh-faced, with big, liquid brown eyes, wonderful skin, and hair that glistened with healthy luster.

I stared at the photo for a while, then flipped through to look at the rest of the pictures. Here were the unpopular girls, with their plump faces, funny hairstyles, glasses, and acne. And here were the popular cheerleaders. Amazed, I paused to stare at a picture of the Homecoming Queen. She wasn't any prettier than I had been!

But she had been petite, at a stage when the boys' growth hadn't yet caught up to the girls'. She had been vivacious, when the boys were unsure of themselves and needed help from the girls if they were to relate to them at all. But most of all, she had been confident, and in that high school era especially, the way a girl carried herself, the way she *acted,* was vital.

I had lacked those vital qualities then—the petiteness, vivacity, confidence. That meant I didn't consider myself pretty, which meant that I hadn't acted pretty, which meant that others didn't consider me pretty either.

I closed the yearbook thoughtfully. Now—at 46—I feel far

more attractive than I ever did as a high schooler. Therefore, because I believe it, I *am*.

I heard similar stories from other women I talked to—regardless of age. Women in their 20s told me they felt prettier, sexier, than they did as teenagers. Women in their 30s believed they were just coming into their own, and they felt that being 33 or 34 put a woman in the prime of her life. One woman of 51, who was astonished to be recommended as sexy for my book, told me that she, too, feels more alluring now than she ever has.

"I look much younger than fifty-one," she told me proudly. "At least, people tell me all the time that I do. And I'm proud of my age, I don't hide it. The other night I was out and I played this game with my date—I bet him he could not guess how old I was. He guessed way young—in the early forties—and I had to show him my driver's license to prove it. He still didn't believe me! I guess I am having an awful lot of fun, I didn't think it could be like this at my age."

Sexy Women Make a Man Feel Desirable as a Male

From an old book called *Fascinating Womanhood* published in the 60s and full of material that would scandalize most feminists, I picked up a tidbit of information that rings with eternal truth. What a man wants you to admire more than anything, author Helen B. Andelin asserts, are his *manly qualities*. It doesn't help to admire traits in a man which are admirable in both men and women, such as honesty, or good sense of humor—because anyone can have those, and the man will be disappointed. It is his masculinity that he wants noticed and admired, and he'll be fascinated by the woman who can help him see himself as virile, desirable, male.[8] (After all, don't we feel the same about men who find us female and desirable?)

I believe that sexy women instinctively sense this important truth about men—that a man wants to feel desirable as a male. More than half of the men I surveyed said that sexy women seem sexually drawn to them "sometimes," and a third said women seem drawn "usually."

A woman's sexual interest in a man heightens his good feelings about himself and makes him extremely receptive to her. The late Marilyn Monroe was a woman who could make a man feel as if he was the only male on earth. Said Billy Travilla, costume designer for *Gentlemen Prefer Blondes,* "She was the one woman I've known who could make a man feel tall, handsome, fascinating . . . you were the king of the evening if she so decided. She made you feel like the only one, even when you were not."[9]

Men told me things like, "I think if a sexy woman is interested in me, I'm going to focus on my own self. In essence it will make me feel more sexy, more desirable."

Agreed a 39-year-old writer, "Sexy women make you feel special, as if they've singled you out because of your irresistible, powerfully masculine charm. The truly sexy women can simultaneously make half a dozen men feel as if each one is the only one she's really interested in. Sexy women also give the feeling that if you play your cards right, they're both available and more than willing. Female sex appeal plays upon the masculine need to feel special and to receive attention."

Sexy Women Subtly Suggest Availability, Even if They Never Act on It

As the male writer above pointed out, a sexy woman makes a man feel that he could "play his cards right" and find her willing—even if this isn't necessarily so.

"They (sexy women) definitely imply that there's more there than just the conversation—maybe not now but if you treat them right . . . a hint of getting together," amplified another man.

Female sexual availability *is* part of the male fantasy, and men like to think that their particular brand of attractiveness is more than sufficient to turn a woman on. But there is a very, very fine line here. As a high school principal pointed out to me, "A man likes to feel that a woman might be coming on very, very strong, but she isn't that way for all men, just for him. It really turns him off if he thinks that she does that for everyone."

How do men feel about women being sexually assertive?

In real life most men prefer the word *subtle* to characterize the feminine approach. Men say things like "She should be gentle in her approach," "She should know how to seduce without seeming that she is seducing," and "Must be ladylike even when she is coming on strong." One study found that 47 percent of the men surveyed agreed with this statement about female aggressiveness: *"If it's done subtly, in a feminine way, it's nice; if in a pushy way, it's a turn-off."*

Sexy women can afford to be more subtle, maybe because they are already emitting sexy "vibes,' so the messages they transmit do not have to be blatant.

I asked women how they showed a man they were interested in him sexually, and what instructions they would give to another woman if she wanted to "come on strong" to a man. Most of the women told me they would be subtle in their approach, trying to read the man first to see if he was interested. "It all depends on the person and how well you know him," said one 24-year-old woman. "You just have to read *him* and how he feels about you sexually. I don't just come out with it, this has never been an issue."

Many women spoke of setting the scene for romance. "Showing you care in little ways," is what one 27-year-old office manager told me she would do. "Doing cuddly, romantic-type things, candlelight things, not necessarily cooking gourmet meals but fixing champagne hors d'oevres, having candlelight, putting pillows on the floor. When you sit on a couch it's more up straight and rigid. Sitting on the floor is more intimate and relaxed, it sets a mood."

Others used casual touching to give the man the idea. "Indicate that you're physically attracted by some kind of touching, a light touch on the arm," instructed one woman. "Make good eye contact. More and more men are offish if you're too pushy."

But apparently pushy also makes it—at least sometimes. Bobbi, one exception to the subtle women I talked to, tends to be flamboyant in her behavior, and has men buzzing in circles around her at the singles group she belongs to. She thoroughly enjoys the attention. "I am very bold and blunt," she told me. "I'd love to take your clothes off you.' Yes, I'd say that. I have to feel real comfortable, though, and in a good mood. Sometimes it works. When I first met Ken, he made me melt. I stayed away from him for about four months, I felt as if he could read my mind. But once the ice was broken, then I could be more my real self. Now, when he comes off the plane to see me, I say, 'Hey! You! Take your clothes off!' "

One researcher has found that preferences for soft- or hard-sell assertiveness divide pretty much along class lines. White-collar and professional men generally prefer the softer, subtler approach. But blue-collar men show an interesting polarity. That is, blue-collar men are almost three times as likely as other classes to feel that aggressiveness is a turn-off, but at the same time working-class men also endorse the hard, sexy sell.[10]

The explanation for this contradiction may be that more blue-collar men view women in the "whore-madonna" syndrome, either as willing sex objects or as pure paragons who wouldn't dream of being too-sexy or crude. If a "nice girl" comes on strong, they'll view it as a turn-off, but if a more sexually liberal woman makes a blunt approach, then it's acceptable.

Not all women can carry off approaching a man with a hard sell. One married male friend wrote me about an incident that happened in a bar. "An attractive, slender brunette sat close to me and insisted on buying me a drink. She made a point of developing eye contact when we spoke and gently caressed my arm and leg during our conversation. I loved every moment of our time together, but I also felt rather guilty. When the woman pointedly massaged my thigh and slipped her hand between my legs, I panicked. (Would a real stud ever admit such a god-awful, shameful response?) A trifle regretfully, I left the bar soon afterward."

Said Dr. Avodah Offit, author of *The Sexual Self and Night Thoughts: Reflections of a Sex Therapist,* "When women who are uncertain about sexuality decide to initiate it, they often act far more aggressively than necessary. It's like using a bulldozer to dig up violets. They haul out this vast machinery to insist on something that would have come very easily otherwise. . . . Being sexually assertive includes being sexually reassuring. Accepting, knowing how to bring a man out sexually, letting a man know that she is interested, cooperative—these are all part of it."[11]

What happens when a woman is perceived by a man as being "too permissive" sexually? This actually erodes an important part of sex appeal, according to several studies that have been done. In one, at Old Dominion University in Norfolk, Virginia, students were asked to rate "permissive" women on various personality qualities. Both men and women rated the permissive woman as more irresponsible, immoral, insecure, and immature than the neutral or more sexually conservative woman. The students did think that permissive women would be friendlier—which figures—but were more likely to want the conservative women as friends. [12]

Success is Sexy

As *Ladies Home Journal* found out, its "sexiest wives," were generally successful at work as well as at a sexual relationship, and two-thirds of them had jobs outside the home, half earning more than $15,000 a year. [13]

Success at doing something, one popular self-help writer advises, is like a sexual aphrodisiac. Any success, from getting a big account to raising a prize show dog, raises a woman's self-esteem and gives her a special glow that transmits itself to others and makes her seem more desirable. One woman told me that it is on the days that she has some hard-won success at work that men turn on to her most. "After I make a sale at work, there is such a good, high feeling. When you talk to any guy, you glow, and this comes off as pretty or sexy."

Men do this all the time, this woman went on to remark. "They have a success, they act confident and they get women. A man who's cocky, very confident in a bar . . . women are drawn to him, attracted to him. He thinks he's attractive and he projects that image, he gets women."

Says Letty Cottin Pogrebin, "It's sexy to be competent. Not silly sexy, like perfume on your kneecaps, but just downright attractive. A self-assured, smart lady executive with a warm smile and a cool head can run rings around a dewy-eyed dumb dumb with a powder puff for a brain. It's enchanting to be able *and* adorable."[14]

Axioms of Sex Appeal

1. An important part of sex appeal is what goes on in the mind. When a woman flirts with a man she should keep in mind two thoughts—first, *his* attractiveness, and secondly, *her own*.

2. Sexual awareness is a very close relative of self-esteem. A woman who feels herself to be sexy, vital, and desirable will be.

3. Sexy women like men and feel that they make good friends, and this genuine liking of males may be one of the secrets of the deep appeal of these women.

4. Sexy women like their bodies, and are pretty well satisfied with the way they look, finding only minor things wrong with themselves. Body-liking is probably another big secret of sex appeal.

5. Sexy women are excellent at making a man feel desired as a male, and in admiring his manly traits. Most of the men I talked to said certain women seem sexually drawn to them. Sexy women subtly suggest availability, even if they never act on it.

6. However, men usually prefer the subtle approach, saying things like the woman "should be gentle," "should know how to seduce without seeming that she is seducing." Sexy women instinctively know this, and in interviews most of them admitted that they seldom send out blatant messages.

7. Success is also sexy, and when a woman has had a triumph at work, this is often transmitted to her attitude, making her glow.

5

The Body Language of Sex Appeal

A maid that laughs is half taken.

—John Ray,
English Proverbs

Do sexy women behave differently? The majority of men over-whelmingly believe that they do! In fact body language, for men, is like a marker that flags out certain women for more detailed scrutiny.

One 37-year-old man told me about a woman he had seen once in a bar who he considered "pure sex." "She wasn't wearing really sexy clothes, nothing overt, she just wore slacks. But she was very, very sexy. She squirmed while standing there, I mean she just slithered. It wasn't conscious, it was just *her*. Mostly the way she moved her torso and legs, it wasn't like a little subtle thing with her hands and feet, it was the whole image, enough to be noticeable to me as a man. I saw her as being a nympho, extremely sexually inclined. She looked very uninhibited."

Most men believe that sexy women do have a flirtacious way of talking and relating to men, use eye contact a lot, and have a provocative way of sitting, standing, walking, etc. Sexy women also touch the men they are talking to, at least sometimes.

One school of men, however, believes that body language is secondary to the physical appeal of the body itself. In other words, if a woman has a sexy body, she doesn't have to act sexy—she already *is*. "It's just that they are built different to begin with," as one 24-year-old man explained to me. "So it doesn't matter. If one of those aspects catches my eye I tend to think of them in those terms. *When you think the woman is sexy you look for actions you think are sexy*."

So what actions are sexy? There is a whole smorgasbord of sexy body language, enough to be covered in two chapters. However, one of the things men told me is that sexy women move *smoothly*. Remember when we were little girls and our mothers admonished us about moving with grace and care?

Sexy women appear to have listened to these lessons. As one man pointed out, "They aren't careless about how they sit/walk/talk, and they would automatically not be sloppy. Sloppy is not sexy."

Agreed another man, "These women are at ease, very smooth when they walk or sit, etc., whether they are at a formal, sit-down dinner, or watching TV in jeans."

Sexy women aren't stuffy, and their movements often project—either obviously or subtly—raw sensuality. Ken, 33, describes a woman he met in a bar. Even though this incident happened several years ago, it's very clear in his mind. "This woman walked in and immediately there were six or seven men surrounding her. She wasn't even that good-looking, she was around 40, but man, could she string them along. She gave me the eye, she's really inviting, it's like, *'I like your looks.'*" She was using that Mae West kind of body language, really projecting sex, like, 'I like you.' It was the most exaggerated type of that thing I've ever seen."

Peter Bogdanovitch discussed Cybill Shepherd's body language when she arrived to audition for *The Last Picture Show*. The actress came in wearing jeans and a jacket, and sat down next to a coffee table where there was a rose in a vase. "She started playing with the rose while she talked—and, like in a cartoon, I expected it to wither from the heat."[1]

Whether it takes place in a bar or in a producer's office, at the office or at a cocktail party, body language telegraphs sex to the male. One of the best ways women use their femaleness is through their walk.

I saw a recent *Geech* cartoon in which two plump matrons in bathing suits are standing by the ocean. One says to the other, "Oh, Nadine, there's a real art to beach strolling."

"There is?"

"Yeah, and it's a lot harder than it sounds. The trick is to walk sexy and look bored."

"I am bored."

"Now comes the hard part. . . ."

Men are inveterate women-watchers, and one of the prettiest things that a woman can do is to stroll past with a certain swingy, free-striding roll of the hips. One 26-year-old lawyer, indeed, was very specific in his insistence that he can only be really turned on by a woman after he watches her walk.

"Walking is most of it," he said. "The most important thing. Kind of a confident walk, snotty, with that kind of look, like, 'I dare you.' Dangerous. Confidence is the thing. If a woman's head is down, if she's got slumped shoulders, she's either in a bad mood or a slouch of a person. But if she moves at a fast pace, with her head up, looking around, that's sexy. She walks right by . . . gives a little smile out of the corner of her mouth, has a way with her eyes. It's not really a swing, it might just be that her feet are a little bit out, this gives a little bounce, a hop in your step. I don't like a swing because it's manufactured. I go to get lunch in Birmingham sometimes, and I sit on a bench and watch the women walk by. Anyone can have a good walk, it can help anyone."

I pressed another man to describe a sexy walk. "Sexy women usually walk sexy," he began. "With a slight wiggle of their ass. They wiggle as if they are trying to consummate penetration for an orgasm."

He was speaking perfectly seriously. The whole interview had been, in fact, on a serious tone, and this was quite a departure.

"Hey, wait a minute," I said. "Do you mean this? Are you sure you aren't putting me on?"

"No, I mean it. I said exactly what I mean. They walk as if they are trying to consummate penetration for an orgasm. They leave you breathless in anticipation of their next move."

All right. Well. . . .

According to one expert on the human gait, the human walk is much more than just locomotion. It can be used as an erotic instrument, much as dance has been used to elicit male sexual response.

The late Florenz Ziegfeld had a format he often used to select the glamorous show girls he used in the Ziegfeld Follies. He would stretch a white screen across a stage and then have the girls, scantily clad and in high heels, strut across the stage behind the screen. Ziegfeld could see only the silhouette of each girl.

He said, "Before I see their faces I want to see how they walk. There's more sex in a walk than in a face, or even in a figure. A woman can have the most beautiful face and the most glorious form. But if the walk isn't exactly right, it can spoil the whole damn thing. Any woman who doesn't take advantage of her feminine asset by learning to walk right, loses a lot of her sex attraction."[2] Legend has it that the late Marilyn Monroe cut a quarter of an inch off one high heel, so that when she walked, her fanny would wiggle enticingly.

Once I attended a large fund-raiser where door prizes were being awarded. There must have been 350 people standing around the edge of that room, all of them with sheafs of door prize tickets in their hands. The woman who'd won a bottle of French wine was what some people call "buxom." She had a round, curvy figure, and her large breasts were high, firm, and undeniably sensuous.

As she walked back from the podium with her bottle of wine, a hush fell upon the room. It was one of those once-in-a-lifetime silences that seem to reverberate, and would have terrified most women I know if they had been its subject. But this was a woman of poise and dignity. Her smooth, flowing, hint-at-sensual walk didn't even falter as she walked back to her place. Her *walk* was so proud and sexy that it turned a potentially embarrassing moment into something quite different.

Watching a Miss World competition last year on television, I was struck at the most notable difference in the young women. All were beautiful, but some, as they approached the camera for their few seconds of glory, walked nervously, almost jerkily, their stride without smoothness. Others were sinuous, seeming almost to flow toward the camera. It was these sinuous young women who, according to the three males with whom I was watching the competition, were the most sexy.

There are several factors that make a feminine walk particularly watchable. One is simply the construction of the female body, which has decreed that our hips are wider than men's, thus affecting the swing of the thighs and producing a more swaying gait. The other, according to William Rossi, our expert on the foot and shoe, has to do with the calf. "The main focus is on the calf," he writes. "Not only its shapely curves but the mobility of the calf muscles beneath. The rhythmic tensing and untensing of these cords, slimming down to the Achilles tendon just above the heel, can hold the eye fascinated. . . ."[3]

In order to pinpoint what makes a gait sexy, let's take a look at the opposite, an unsexy walk. During a recent hospitalization, I had a chance to observe hospital patients tottering down the hall, clinging to a wall railing and doing what a friend of mine calls the "Crittenton Shuffle." This wide-legged, cautious, infirm walk is as far down the spectrum from sexy as it's possible to get.

William Rossi has studied the female walk extensively, and says that a "desexed" walk occurs when the person places her feet far apart to widen the base for more security in walking. Who walks this way? The aged, the very obese, patients in hospitals, pregnant women in their eighth and ninth months. In fact, Rossi insists, a sign of advancing age and declining sexiness in a woman is when her gait changes. She loses springiness in her step, walks with her feet wider apart, and toes out.

The average woman, some experts say, strides with her feet approximately three to five inches apart from each other. If her feet are any wider apart than that, the gait is less sexy. If they are closer together, the walk is far *more* sexy.

A sexy walk could be created then, by pretending that you were trying to walk a chalk line. With each step one foot crosses just slightly over the other, forcing a slightly exaggerated swing of the hips and buttocks. This is the model's walk, the swingy, sexy strut practiced by showgirls and others who must transmit a natural sensuousness.

But even if we aren't models and don't want to exaggerate to that extent, we can still add to our appeal in another way—by throwing our shoulders back and thrusting our chests out proudly. I was always self-conscious about my large breasts, developing a permanent, protective "hunch" to hide my size. I was enrolled in a dance class and one day the instructor took me aside.

"Julia," she began, "You're too self-conscious about your breasts. Walk straight and proud and stick them out rather than hunching forward. You won't believe this, but that is actually going to make them look much smaller, rather than larger. You're going to look a whole lot better, and thinner, too." I no longer remember all the jazz steps she taught me, but that proud walk has become part of my body repertoire.

The wearing of high heels also adds to the flavor of the sexy walk, because it restricts the woman's stride, requiring her to use smaller, sexier steps. The reason for this goes back centuries into the darker recesses of human history. It is related most especially to fetter and bondage. Some males have found it erotic to view the woman as restricted in her movements, helpless, dependent and at their mercy. This may not be on a conscious level (to give men credit) but the thoughts may nonetheless exist.

"Stepping chains" were worn in ancient Palestine by nubile young slave girls, to limit the length of their stride and make it sexier. (We still see remnants of this custom in the slave ankle bracelets some women wear.) And of course there was foot-binding in old China, which curtailed the female walk into a small-step, mincing, tottering gait.

Some tribal women in Africa were fitted with knobbed, clog-like sandals that forced them into taking tiny steps. And Japanese women, in their tight-fitting kimonos, were forced into taking delicate, short steps as well. In America, there are tight skirts, and high heels to produce the same effect.

Sitting behavior is another way in which sexy women distinguish themselves from the average. A sexy woman has a re-laxed, self-confidence about her body, and this transmits itself to the way she sits. She isn't tight, but neither is she so loose that her style of sitting totally resembles a man's. According to what men told me, she would tend to sit closer to a man than the "average" woman, and might even move her chair to be more comfortable when talking to him.

Rock star Tina Turner is a prime example of the uninhibited way some sexy women sit. She made this impression on interviewer Mick Farren: "While she talks she is constantly in motion. She stabs with long, blood-red fingernails when she wants to emphasize a point. She is continuously fixing, re-fixing, and generally playing with her amazing honey hair. She uses the couch in the hotel suite like some kind of gymnastic device. She swivels, she pulls her legs under herself, at one point she is almost in a full lotus position."[4]

I asked one 29-year-old dentist how a sexy woman would sit. He was intrigued by the question. "She'd probably sit across from you fairly close," he responded. "She might have her legs spread slightly, or be sitting in a way that is not confined to society's norms for sitting, but is comfortable for her. I've been to Detroit Athletic Club parties where men and women sat with the chairs pulled up close, so that they were eye to eye, nose to nose. It's sexy if she can sit more freely, as she likes, whether it's cross-legged, or she just brings her legs up and crosses them."

Much has been written on the body language of crossed legs. For instance, if a woman crosses her feet at the ankles, this is receptive language, implying that it's all right for others to approach. If, on the other hand, she crosses her legs high and tight, locking her thighs together, she is shutting people out, being "closed-exclusive."[5]

When a man and a woman are at a party getting to know each other, they may position themselves to block out others by using their arms to close a circle, by crossing their feet toward each other, or by leaning toward each other. And of course there is the ages-old leg-crossing ploy . . . that is, the woman with silken grace keeps crossing and recrossing her legs, each time revealing a slight hint of thigh, perhaps even subtly touching or playing with her knees or thighs.[6]

I saw one sexy woman posing for a photograph with her boyfriend. She sat with her legs conventionally crossed, but just before the photographer snapped the picture, she tugged at the hem of her dress, pulling it high enough to reveal just her kneecaps. The photo shows a charming, smiling woman giving just a tiny, half-teasing leg show.

All the pretty behavior of crossing legs, adjusting a flirty hem, shifting positions, can be extremely alluring to the male. A poet-in-residence at a university talked to *Psychology Today* about the openly seductive behavior of his women students. "The girls come into my office flashing their thighs, wriggling about in the chair, talking about poetry. Perhaps they're doing what nature tells them to do. Perhaps they don't know what they're doing. But I know—and I notice it."[7]

Sitting is only one way in which sexy women are more relaxed. As one man told me, "Sexy women do little things like take their shoes half off and play with their feet. They curl their toes and do things like that, and the body language of their feet says, 'I am sensual.' "

The act of taking off the shoes in the company of others can be interpreted by men as receptivity to intimate action. We have already seen that feet are a sexy, erogenous zone, and numbers of men do find feet stimulating. Whether we agree with his interpretation or not, one male judge in an attempted sexual assault case said, "When a woman kicks off her shoes in the private company of a man, it's a suggestive act of undressing."

Controlling Body Language by Opposites

At a party the talk turned to sex appeal, and several woman wanted to talk about flirting. "I don't flirt, and I know I don't," a pretty 33-year-old woman announced. "When I am talking to a man it's as if there is this sheath of ice all around me. But it's funny . . . why do I have so many homosexual friends?"

Another woman, a bit older, said she didn't flirt either. "I'm always astonished when a man says I've been doing it. I remember when I was married, it was as if I walked around in a kind of a cloud, I just wasn't aware of things like that. If a man was coming on to me I didn't even realize it, and yet my husband got very angry several times at men making advances toward me. He actually got to the point where he was grabbing up these men by the scruff of the neck. I was totally bewildered. I hadn't even realized they were coming on to me that way. And now that I'm single, I still get people who tell me I act as if I were married. I feel awkward and ridiculous, trying to put on an act. Is it possible to train people to flirt?"

As these women have suggested, the most difficult thing about body language is that most of it is unconscious—we don't *know* that we are doing things, we just do them or not do them. Most of the women that I talked to about sex appeal admitted to me that they don't really know everything they do because much of it "just happens." And the men, too, were often unable to pinpoint *exactly* how a sexy woman might flirt with them—they just knew she did.

But necessity forces some women to face their own unconscious actions. Active in the business world, or pursued by many men and obviously unable to have relationships with all of them, they have learned to screen their body language very effectively, mostly to say no. And this brings up a very interesting point. *Any woman who is able to use her body to say no, can turn that behavior around to say yes, just as effectively.*

First, we need to realize just what the difference is between

warm and cold behavior. Early in my marriage I was totally un-
aware of body signals and their meaning. One night my husband
and I had gone to a dull party. He was talking with other people,
I didn't know many of the guests and quickly grew bored. When
a man approached me and began talking to me, I stuck with
him because it seemed easier than trying to circulate. We must
have spent nearly two hours chatting while I stifled my wish
to be elsewhere. At 2 AM I was relieved to go home, and I completely forgot my party partner.

However, he didn't forget me. I received my comeuppance
the following Monday morning when two events occurred: First,
the man telephoned to invite me to lunch. I was totally
shocked—both of us were married and I didn't have the slightest
desire for such a liason. But then, a few minutes later, came
the second surprise, a phone call from our hostess, who cattily
informed me that the man's wife had been jealous because I
had talked to him for so long!

Red-faced, I hung up from the second call realizing that I
had brought all this on myself by spending far too much time
talking to one man. Apparently prolonged talking to a man—
more than twenty minutes or so—is a sign of sexual interest,
and men take it that way.

What kind of behavior in a woman does show liking—or
disliking? This was the question put to college students at the
University of Illinois at Urbana by a group of researchers. Behaviors these students rated as "warmest," included:

> smiles frequently
> has a happy face
> works her eyes from his head to his toes
> looks into his eyes
> moves toward him
> touches his hand
> smiles with mouth open
> sits directly facing him

The "coldest" behaviors they named included these:

> gives a cold stare
> looks at the ceiling

sneers

cleans her fingernails

frowns

chain smokes

moves away from him

gives a fake yawn[8]

Nadine is a single woman in her 30s, who has been unconsciously using "cold" body language to keep men at a distance from her. I met Nadine at a Tupperware party. Nadine is a shy-looking blonde with reserved mannerisms, and, in fact, when she first saw me she stared at me almost suspiciously, inspecting me carefully. But as the party progressed, gradually Nadine relaxed. As she did so, her face began to light up, giving her a pretty, open, vulnerable look that hadn't been apparent at first.

We were talking about this book, which I was then researching, and Nadine kept frowning, looking troubled.

Finally she leaned forward. "I really need to know how to flirt," she announced. "I don't know how anymore. I go to cocktail parties and I get so turned off. I get tired of sitting around, so I go up and talk to a man and he doesn't seem very interested, he moves away the first chance he gets." She shrugged half-angrily. "What am I supposed to do? There's something wrong. I just can't flirt anymore."

As I talked with her I learned something of Nadine's story. She had had two marriages, both to substance abusers. Both men had been sweet and attentive, lavishing attention upon her—until after the marriage. Then things changed. "When my second husband started barking out orders to me, telling me, 'Go sit down over there and shut up,' I was like, *God.* This can't be happening. It can't be."

Now divorced, Nadine is terrified that the same thing will happen to her again.

"I just can't flirt anymore," she repeated anxiously.

"But you did flirt on that boat cruise," a girlfriend, who had been sitting nearby, interrupted. "Remember that waiter—Nello or whatever his name was? Remember how he looked at you? He liked you."

Nadine's face softened. "He kept bringing my food," she explained, "and my friends would poke me and say, 'Hey, he's looking at you.' And I'd say, 'Oh, go on with you.' But one day I turned around and he *was* staring at me and I . . . " She laughed. "I almost died, because they were right! After that I started talking to the guy and we had a great time."

"And remember last weekend?" the friend prompted. "Those two guys we met . . . ?"

Nadine shifted, looking more and more troubled. "I didn't do anything special," she qualified. "Besides those two guys were married. And Nello . . . yes, I did see him on the cruise, but that was all."

Nadine's case is a typical example of unconsciously selective flirting. She *is* perfectly capable of flirting, but only with men who are "safe," i.e., married, or who she knows she will never see again.

Actually, there are two Nadines. One is the reserved, almost suspicious woman I was introduced to, the Nadine who is cautious about getting to know new people for fear they will hurt her. Nadine wasn't trying to be this way, she just was, but the message came through to *me* loud and clear. If I picked up on it, why wouldn't the men with whom she comes in contact? Nobody wants to flirt with a suspicious person. Suspicion is the very antithesis of flirting.

The second Nadine is the relaxed one, the one who has decided she likes you, whose face lights up when she speaks, and who projects a vulnerable prettiness. It is this Nadine who was able to flirt on the boat cruise, who laughed with the two married men, *who was able to flirt.*

On the other hand, skilled flirters know when they are turning a man on. Their flirting isn't always deliberate, but more a matter of accurate instinct.

Anne is in her mid-30s, a bubbly, likeable redhead who was better able than most women to articulate her flirting methods. Anne placed an ad in a singles' column. She got about 75 letters and interviewed approximately two dozen of these men. "It was a crazy experience, because some of the men were excessively romantic, and really wanted to pursue a relationship— like, they were ready to get started right then. Or they'd actually ask me, 'Well, what about it? Are we going to have a relationship?'

"There must be a lot that goes on unconsciously with flirting, because whenever I really didn't like the guy, somehow I'd project this. If I didn't like him I would shorten the time we spent together with some excuse. I would look around the room a lot more, fiddle with the menu more, not look directly into his eyes. I wouldn't act as interested in him; I wouldn't ask as many really good questions about him. I'd talk about hobbies instead of *him*. I wouldn't be as open, I'd be much more casual and superficial. I think I even sneaked a few looks at my watch, I'm ashamed to say."

I asked Anne what she did when she was interested in the man. It turns out that she did the exact *opposite*. "Oh, if I liked him a lot I would lean forward and look him right in the eyes when we talked, I wasn't looking around the room at all. I'd casually take my glasses off, to show him what my eyes looked like without the glasses. I'd talk about him a lot more. I'd just be very relaxed, I'd laugh more, I wasn't in a hurry to leave, I'd maybe accidently brush his arm or touch him to emphasize a point."

Using these methods Anne did meet one man that she especially liked, and she ended up having a relationship with him. Anne *knew how* to show positive interest, and when Ben happened along, it wasn't even a matter of technique—Anne just did what came naturally.

When a woman knows what she is doing negatively, and is able to "turn off" men at will, then it's easy to turn that behavior around to draw men to her. Women who attend singles functions quickly learn to get control of their body language to encourage or discourage. Pat, 30, told me that when her date leaves to go to the restroom, she uses a technique to discourage other men from coming up to her table while he is gone. "I sit facing the wall usually, not making eye contact with anyone— this keeps the other guys off. Now, if I did want someone to come up to me, I'd do just the opposite. I'd sit looking out at the room, looking at people, with a fairly happy and comfortable expression on my face."

Another woman, Lana, accidentally discovered a turn-off technique when her girlfriend insisted on meeting her for a drink in a nearby bar-lounge. "When I got there it turned out to be a singles bar. Well, I hadn't bargained on that. I was afraid my boyfriend would get mad at me if he found I'd gone to a singles bar, so I stood there looking down at the formica bar top. I didn't want to get picked up and I didn't. But my girlfriend was acting just the opposite because she did want to meet someone. She was looking all around her, laughing a lot, acting really sparkly, and several men came up to talk to her."

Experts in the field of sexual harrassment at work give women advice on how to avoid unwanted advances. Many women complain that they are not being taken seriously at work and attempt, through dress and behavior, to "tone down" the sexual overtones that take place at every level when men and women interact. Still, these days, sex *has* entered the workplace, and there are women who do want to flirt, or more, while on the job. Further, as one working woman points out, "In this day and age, when half the population is single or divorced, and everyone's in the work force—looking and wanting—that's where people meet. They meet in the office."

Here is what one book advises women to do if they want to avoid being harrassed on the job.[9] Also, note what happens when we reverse the rules and do the *opposite:*

Follow a business dress code. This means dressing in a standard business outfit of skirted suit and contrasting blouse, of the type recommended by John T. Malloy in *The Woman's Dress For Success Book.* Staid, safe, and dull.

Doing the opposite: But if a woman does want to attract male attention on the job or off, then she should *avoid* looking too businessy, and concentrate on wearing a dress, less formal suit, or more feminine attire. As one man put it, "I hate it when a woman wears all black to work. To me that is a "power" suit and not very appealing at all."

Adopt professional behavior. That is, don't talk about details of your personal life to the men around you, but steer the conversation to the work at hand. Talk about work, not you and him. That will nip any flirting behavior in the bud.

Doing the opposite: But if you *do* want to appear sexier, then obviously the more you can talk about the personal, the better.

Steer conversation away from work toward personal things, and confide in the man about some of your problems, concerns, fears, etc. Lannie, 34, newly separated, just got a job as a word processor and talks about herself to almost everyone at work. She tells co-workers her personal problems, concerns, and humorous worries. As a result she has built up a circle of social acquaintances at work, even giving a party for about 25 of them and receives regular lunch invitations from men.

Create a male protector. In other words, invent a ficticious boyfriend or husband if you don't have one, in order to keep matters on an impersonal level. Your mythical male will serve as a barrier to unwanted attentions.

Doing the opposite: But if you'd rather appear sexy at work, the opposite will work much better—that is, *don't* talk about your current relationship or husband, because this will make you seem much more available. And never ask about his wife or girlfriend either. In fact, act as if both of you had no attachments whatsoever.

This is what Janice has done at work in her situation with Rob, who is a supervisor in her office. Janet never mentions her live-in boyfriend, pretending he doesn't exist. As a result Rob and others have shown a flirtacious interest in her, and Janice is faced with a dilemma: Should she pursue any of these relationships?

Don't drink alone with him. This gives a man the idea that he's on a date with you, instead of having a business contact. And anything that smacks of dating is a no-no if you want to appear aloof.

Doing the opposite: Naturally, if you do have designs on the man, what better way to enthrall him than with a tete-a-tete alone? Having drinks alone is a good opportunity for plenty of eye contact, flirting, and other "come-close" body language. Jill, on a training seminar with 150 other salesmen, spotted a man she'd like to know better. When others who were drinking with them left, Jill lingered. She and Gregg stayed in the bar until it closed, then adjourned to a nearby all-night coffee shop. The message Jill was sending to Gregg was very clear—her interest in him was not business.

❧ *Talk about his family, meet or befriend his wife, and ask about his wife and kids a lot.* As above, this technique lets a man know that you know he is unavailable, and erects a barrier between you.

❧ Doing the opposite: But if you want matters to go more romantically, the opposite ploy is the one you want to try. That is, never ask about the wife or kids, assuming the fantasy that the man is unattached. Sandi has been carrying on a flirtation with a married man in her office for several years. As she told me, "Ed doesn't want to feel guilty when he's talking to me, so I never bring up his family. Somehow it's just better when we don't talk about real-life problems, such as the fact that he has four kids under the age of twelve. I guess you could say it's sexier that way."

❧ *Refuse lunches or dinners that are "pleasure" and not related to business.* A woman who wants to keep things on a professional level is alert to anything that smacks of a date, and will avoid such situations.

❧ Doing the opposite: Do accept lunch or dinner invitations, knowing that such acceptances signal availability in other areas. Kelli has met several men at work, and regularly accepts invitations to lunch. To her the large company she works for represents a wide pool of available men, and, as she puts it, "Why shouldn't I take advantage? I work nine hours a day, with a one-hour commute each way and I don't have time to go out looking. If I don't meet someone at work, I don't meet him at all."

❧ *Don't ask for or offer to do special favors.* Any time favors are accepted, reciprocity is implied.

❧ Doing the opposite: Asking a man to do you "favors" is a very effective flirting ploy that shows interest on your part, and certainly implies, at minimum, a good friendship.

Flirting is an Art and a Skill

Flirting is a "body language skill," practiced by women in all cultures, all over the globe, from sophisticated Americans to stone-age tribeswomen. Anthropologist David B. Givens points out a fundamental difference between flirtation and seduction. Both, he says, consist of intimate, sexually loaded relations, but "flirtation may be coy and less serious than courtship, while seduction may represent condensed or 'collapsed' courtship, or a quickly resolved version of it."[10]

Most of the people I talked to differentiated between different types of flirting. For instance, there's regular flirting and "serious flirting." "When I flirt seriously," one woman said, "There's a big difference. A man can tell. The difference is inside me. I can't pinpoint it, but I know I'm shier when I flirt seriously."

As another woman pointed out to me, nonserious flirting occurs when the woman "really doesn't care." "I've seen that a lot at dances," she said. "When the women are coming on really strong with their sex appeal, they're flirting outrageously, because all they're out for is a one-night stand. They don't want anything more, so it really doesn't matter, and they can pull out all the stops, dare anything they please. But when you get past that, when you do care, when the man is important to you, then you want to be more discreet when you are flirting."

At a discussion group, quickly the group came to agreement: Types of flirting vary according to the degree of "safeness." Married flirting depends on a barrier of safety. "I like flirting," said one married, sexy woman. "Especially when the other person knows it's for fun, or if they ever asked me to go any farther I wouldn't—except for my mother's doctor in Cleveland."

Several women said that when they were married, they flirted a great deal, in a harmless way, but now that they are single they are much more cautious.

"It was fun; I did it all the time," said one woman, "I loved it. I would flirt with married men and they'd flirt back with me, sometimes I'd even flirt with them in front of their wives. But as soon as I became single, that all changed. Suddenly those barriers were down, anything could happen, and it wasn't safe anymore."

"There is definitely a barrier," agreed a man. "I know at my office it is the married people who flirt most, and you see the single men, they're just going about their business. When you are single, there is nothing to stop you and I think that is what the barrier is. It's a barrier you don't want to go over unless you want something more to happen."

Males react to flirting in one of several ways: Either the man is interested and intrigued, in which case, if he is in a singles bar he may approach the woman, talk to her, lean toward her or move closer. He might ask her to dance, touch, or even kiss her. However, if the man isn't interested he "pretends" not to notice and doesn't flirt back. Sometimes, he gets spooked by some too-overt aggressiveness in the woman, and actually flees the scene.

Studies have been done on flirting behavior with interesting results. One woman who taught classes on flirting in Seattle, Washington, researched the topic and then went out to the lounges and watering holes of Seattle to put her theories into action. "The most surprising thing I found," she told a newspaper later, "was not that most men don't know how to flirt. I expected that. The shocker is, most men don't know when a woman is flirting with them. Ninety-nine percent of guys in their 20s, 30s, and 40s take one look at a woman who is putting out her most obvious signals, gulp, and look back down into their drinks."

It was the men age 50 and older, she maintained, who were best at picking up signals.[11]

Another researcher once visited more than 100 singles bars in order to study flirting signals given off by women, and he also estimated that 85 percent of the men "couldn't tell" when a woman was flirting with them.

But when I told these stories to a man of my acquaintance, he offered a solid explanation for this phenomenon. Simply: "They're not interested. That's why they didn't flirt. Why should they flirt with just anyone? If a man is interested, he's going to respond somehow."

Another study on flirting was done by Monica Moore, Ph.D., at the University of Missouri-St. Louis. She and her co-workers spent 100 hours observing 200 white women, about 18 to 35 years old, all unaccompanied by a man and in a singles-bar setting with at least 25 other people around. Watching each woman for at least half an hour, they monitored flirting signals ranging from smiling to skirt hiking to flirty glances.

One question Moore wanted to answer was whether there

was more flirting activity in a singles-bar setting than there would be, for instance, in a university snack bar or a library. She found, to no one's surprise, that women in the singles bars averaged more than 70 flirting acts per hour, compared to 19 in the snack bar, 10 in the library, and 5 in a women's center meeting.

And the most encouraging finding of all: "Those women who signaled often were also those who were most often approached by men."[12]

How *does* a woman get past a man's barriers, and with her body language get a man to notice her and be intrigued? More on flirting in the next chapter as we delve into a varied selection of flirting techniques.

Axioms of Sex Appeal

1. A woman's body language, for men, is like a marker that flags out certain females for more detailed scrutiny. Many women project a certain type of "raw sensuality" by their body language, whether it be conscious or unconscious.

2. Sexy women are smooth-moving, not careless about how they sit/walk/talk, and they would automatically not be sloppy.

3. A sexy walk is a confident one, and can be an erotic instrument. According to Florenz Ziegfeld, "Any woman who doesn't take advantage of her feminine asset by learning to walk right, loses a lot of her sex attraction."

4. An *unsexy* walk is wide-legged, the feet placed far apart to widen the base for more security in walking. To stride with the feet about three to five inches apart from each other is about average. If you bring the feet any closer than that, sexiness increases.

5. High heels are sexier than flat shoes because of the actual physical changes that high heels make in the way a woman carries her body, and because of a subtle, unconscious flavor of "fetter and bondage."

6. A sexy woman sits in a loose, free, relaxed, self-confident way, and she also tends to sit closer to a man than a nonsexy woman.

7. There are many small, pretty gestures of leg-crossing, or taking the shoes off in the company of others, that show sexiness or receptivity.

8. Much body language is unconscious, and therefore hard for a woman to direct, until she learns to control her body language by opposites. Knowing what she does to *turn off* men can help a woman learn to undo those particular gestures and turn men back on again. Any woman who is able to use her body to say no, can turn that behavior around to say yes.

9. Women need to learn the differences between "warm" and "cold" behavior. Being suspicious is the very antithesis of flirting.

10. There are certain behaviors, such as following a business dress code, never talking about personal things, creating a male protector, or refusing nonbusiness lunches or dinners, that will keep a woman from being sexually harrassed at work. But if a woman does want attention from males at work (or anywhere else) she should do the opposite of these things.

11. There are many different types of flirting, some recreational, and others "serious." These vary according to the degree of safety the participants feel. Males react to flirting in three ways. Either they are interested, they "pretend" not to notice, or they get spooked and leave the scene.

12. Women who "signal" with their body language most often are the most likely to be approached by men.

6

The Secrets of Flirting

*When a woman looks right into my
eyes and holds the look, I know she's
interested.*

—Male interviewee

The scene is "Nickey's," a popular singles watering hole. A rock band plays a heavy rhythmic beat, while hordes of men and women between the ages of 21 and 40 mill around a long bar, laughing, jostling, moving from one conversation group to another. They eye each other, approach, consider, reject, make connections.

The bar is alive with flirting language, and these 200 or so people are all sending out bodily signals—as many as 70 per hour each.

Flirting, as I mentioned in Chapter 5, is a very complex phenomenon; scientists have isolated up to 52 separate behaviors, some as small as the lift of an eyebrow or shrug of a shoulder.

Anthropologist David P. Givens has researched flirting behaviors in detail, both in animals and humans. Animals, he says, have two basic goals that must be accomplished in sexual preliminaries—or mating can't take place at all. First, the female has to show that she's not going to be aggressive, a real danger in many species equipped with fangs and claws. Second, the male must overcome her aversion to physical contact. [1]

What does all of this mean for the female mammal? To mate, she has to convince the male that she is safe, that she won't be aggressive, which means that she must display "submissive" behavior. And anyone who has ever owned a dog has seen plenty of examples of submissive animal behavior.

The adult male and female mammal often perform maternal-infant behaviors to signal they are ready to form sexual attachments, such as jaw-nuzzling, snout-licking, grooming, caressing, and playing. Interestingly, Givens says, when animals are submissive, they revert to babyish behaviors, and the same is true for humans as well. Many so-called flirting behaviors can be observed in the nursery school between two tots who are trying to get acquainted!

Human beings apparently are influenced by their biological past. Like antelopes, elephants, or wild dogs, the human male needs the biological assurance that the woman he covets *is* approachable, and won't be aggressive.

Certain characteristics of human females, such as relative hairlessness, smooth complexion, and soft voice may contribute to this easing of the male apprehensions. And it is undoubtedly no accident that many men in my survey listed as turn-offs women who are too "pushy" or aggressive. Non-submissive body language may be a sexual turn-off.

Shoulder shrugging is a culturally wide submissive behavior reported as early as 1872 by Charles Darwin. Other submissive actions (no doubt a surprise to many women who consider themselves liberated and free) include tilting the head, raising or flexing the shoulders, and clasping or holding one's own body, such as holding the upper arms or forearms, or joining the hands. Eye-contact, followed by averting the gaze downward, is important submission-type behavior.

Researchers have discovered, by observing flirting couples in cafeterias and other settings, that what they say verbally, isn't nearly as important as what they say with their bodies. Maintains Givens, who observed this for himself, "Even a highly technical scientific or political discussion, from a nonverbal point of view, can be carried on flirtaciously."[2]

In fact, one woman with aggressive feminist views came to Dr. Givens with a problem: Although she had assertive things to say, men were coming on to her sexually. This woman, let's call her Terri, had assumed what Givens called a habitual or chronically flirtacious pose.

Dr. Givens made an hour-long video tape of Terri having a spirited argument about feminist issues with a male friend. Verbally, the argument was lively and sometimes profane. But nonverbally, Givens discovered, Terri's body language was extremely meek and submissive, seductively so, in sharp contrast to the strong verbal message she was trying to transmit.

"The woman behaved in a courting-like manner throughout the conversation," Givens related in a scientific article. "Lengthy periods of smiling-facing-gaze alternating with downward eye aversion were used. The head was held habitually in a laterally tilted position while listening and speaking, and shoulder-flexing/supinating was conspicuously evident."[3]

"Supinating," as used here, incidentally, means to rotate the hand or forearm so that the surface of the palm is upward.

Terri also spoke in a soft, somewhat high voice, and even when arguing, she engaged in such sexy, submissive behaviors as stretching, smiling, preening the hair, and cocking the head.

After she viewed her own tape and learned what behaviors were causing men to respond in a sexual way, Terri was able to eliminate these unconsciously sexy behaviors and discourage advances she did not want. In other words, she got control of her own sex appeal. Another woman might have wished to emphasize these behaviors to make herself more sexy, not less.

Dr. Givens observed another woman who had very good control over her seductiveness. He regularly visited a university cafeteria to study flirtations, and on one visit saw a couple having coffee together after a history class, apparently for the first time. The woman, about 25, would stare into the man's eyes, then lower her own eyes. She smiled abundantly, and made numerous shoulder-shrugging movements. She constantly touched herself, clasped her hands, covered her mouth, touched her cheek. Evidently this flirty body language was highly successful, for Dr. Givens noticed the woman writing down her phone number for the man.

After the man had left, the young woman adopted what Givens calls a socially neutral pose. That is, her face went blank, the animation left it, her shoulders relaxed, and she stopped touching herself. Leaving the cafeteria, she happened to pass in front of a watchful man who was seated at a nearby table. Now her demeanor changed.

"She gazed at him and—in a turnabout, nonflirtacious performance—assumed an unfriendly pose by maintaining the deadpan expression rather than smiling, averting the gaze to the side, and showing the tongue. Blank-faced stare, lateral gaze cut-off, and tongue show may be interpreted as socially negative cues," says Givens, "As indications that a performer would be less than eager to interact."[4]

Individual Components of Flirting

Flirting consists of a number of separate behaviors, some conscious and some unconscious. Some are used almost universally, others occasionally, or only in certain situations. I'll list flirting behaviors in order of most common use.

Smiling. "A maid that laughs is half taken," is the quotation at the beginning of Chapter 4, and abundant smiling, says anthropologist Givens, is a strong and obvious component of flirting. Studies reveal that smiling is one of the most often used signals. Sexy women I've observed flirting do a *lot* of smiling, and this was mentioned over and over by the women I talked to.

I received a lesson in smiling one afternoon from a professional photographer when I was getting my picture taken for a publicity photo. Dmitri LaZaroff has taken photos of many prominent Detroit celebrities, including the Fords, and carefully he instructed me how to "make love to the camera."

He told me, "Let the smile touch your lips just a little, not a large smile that shows the teeth, just a little smile that touches the corner of your lips and shows in your eyes." The result was a softly seductive picture, one of my favorites, with a come-hither smile that I have since used in flirting with (often) devastating effect.

"I really like to flirt," one vibrant woman of 29 told me. "How do you flirt? I think being really positive, not a real fake, but smiling, energetic. . . . Laugh a lot, come up positive. When a guy is at a singles dance, he's going to ask the girls to dance that have a smile on their faces, who are smiling even though they don't feel like smiling on the inside."

Eye Contact. This is the second most important element in flirting, mentioned by all the women I interviewed, and most of the men. In fact, when I surveyed 73 men, nearly all of them said that a sexy woman looks them in the eye either "nearly always" or "usually." Eye contact is vital to flirting!

As Julius Fast points out, there is a "moral looking time" in eye contact. If a woman holds a man's glance even a fraction of a second past that point, then the message she's transmitting is very clear—she's interested.

There are all different kinds of eye-looks. One of the most effective shows the necessary "submission." This is when a woman looks into a man's eyes, then lowers her own, as if in shyness. In his book, *The Human Animal: The Mystery of Man's Behavior,* Hans Hass discusses the basic movements of flirtation, which he says are common all over the world among many cultures. The sequence is simple. The woman gives the man a "smile of provocation or invitation, followed by a 'bashful' lowering of the eyes, a turning away, withdrawal, and apparent tendency toward flight. Visual contact is then resumed and the ambivalent motor sequence may be repeated."[5]

In singles bars, studies have found that one of the most often used eye-looks is the room-encompassing glance, where the woman allows her eyes to sweep the room, making it plain she's looking around for something—or someone—to happen.

Frequent looks are another way of flirting. Said one man, "Sexy women look at you all the time. I picked up on a woman last night at the discussion group I went to; she looked at me every time I spoke, and then she came and sat next to me on the couch."

Then there is the sidelong, or darting glance. This is when the woman steals a glance at a man and—before his eyes can move to lock with hers—she looks away. According to Desmond Morris, this is used as a sign of shyness (another way of being submissive.) The message sent is, 'I am too frightened to look straight at you, but I can't help staring."[6]

"They look at you," explained a controller for a power company. "And not in a way to say, 'There's something wrong,' but it's an approving look. They keep it long enough to look approval and catch you looking, then they look away to let you know they're afraid to let you know they like you, there's a barrier. When they'll allow you to know they like you, it takes away the fear of rejection you have in not knowing what they're thinking."

Bedroom eyes are the opposite of furtive—heavy-lidded, a sleepy, calculating, or appraising look.

"I saw this woman in a bar called *Players,*" says a male friend of mine. "She was surrounded by five guys, and every once in a while she'd look up and give this look: 'I want to go to bed with you.' It was so strong you could just feel it."

The distant, riveting glance is another very effective ploy. Here a woman notices a man from afar, making this fact very, *very* apparent. Usually the two are strangers, and the woman's eye contact rivets the man, drawing his interest magnetically. "You're standing at a party somewhere," one man paints the scene. "You walk past her and you want a second glance. You think you're far away from her, you're standing back to back with her, and then you turn and meet her eyes and she's looking back at you. That's sexy."

One man, David, tells about being wedged in a phone booth on the UCLA campus making a phone call when a coed walked by and gave him a long, long, sizzling look that was "unmistakable" because of its duration, and the slightly suppressed smile that went along with it. David hung up the phone in mid-sentence, rushed out of the booth and caught up to the girl. Their flirtation and eye games lasted several hours; it led to a three-year, live-in relationship.

Then there is the frank, look-him-over glance. For generations, men have eyed women, giving them the up-and-down, not-missing-a-thing sexual onceover that says "I like what I see." Now more women are using this same technique with devastating effectiveness. Several generations ago, Mae West had the look down pat. A writer for *Silver Screen* wrote about the actress: "She gave him the Westian eye business—down on his shoes, his ankles . . . now on his third waistcoat button, now his tie . . . the eyes . . . that's the sexiest eyetrick in the world, if you really want to know. Marlene Dietrich's left to right eye shift is like a bottle of sarsaparilla in an absinthe shop compared with it."[7]

Said one man I interviewed, "Women accuse men of undressing them with their eyes, but men perceive that of women, too. If a woman looked at a man that way, if she was looking him over, say, from ankles to head, her body language can be picked up. Certainly that move is very seductive."

The one-on-one glance, where a woman gazes deeply into a man's eyes, is also strongly sexy. Studies have shown that when people are deeply interested in each other, their pupils actually dilate. One woman told me about a date she had where she and the man stared deeply into each other's eyes. The man's pupils had dilated so much that his eyes looked nearly black.

"Generally I look men right in the eye," said Kathy, a 33-year-old woman who attracts more than her share of male attention. "I have very expressive eyes. 'You talk with your eyes,' men tell me or, 'I love the way your eyes move.' When I get real serious, my eyes go back and forth; I'm looking into their eyes and trying to read what they think of me."

However, prolonged eye contact is difficult for some to maintain, and one woman confessed to me that she sometimes stares at a man's face near the eyes, rather than at the eyes themselves.

Touching. Touching is another strong element of flirtation. The men I polled agreed that sexy women do touch them during the course of a conversation, with about half saying the women do this "nearly always" or "usually," the rest "sometimes." The women, too, agreed: They will often casually touch the man to make a conversational point.

"You use small touches, you touch their shoulder, arm, or hand," said one 27-year-old office manager. "I'm a touchy feely person even with my girlfriends, I establish contact through touch."

Another woman agreed. "I do touch: for instance if they say something funny, I'll pat them on the cheek and say, 'Gee, you're cute.'"

Touching is powerful business, for studies have shown that being touched changes people's moods, making them feel happier, warmer, and more satisfied—even more willing to tip waitresses. Said one businessman, "When I am out at a business lunch I can look around me at the other tables full of business people, they'll be mostly men, and the waitress will look around to see which one of them is going to pay the check. Then she'll touch that person. Every time she comes back to the table she'll touch that person. And she gets bigger tips that way. It works."

Being a "touching" person probably does enhance a woman's appeal to men, while being a nontoucher erects barriers. Glenna has what some people call an abrasive personality. She is crusty, a bit standoffish, and if you say something, she's likely to disagree. She can be almost too assertive—and yet beneath it all you sense the soft interior, the vulnerabilities she's trying to hide.

I like Glenna, but Ed admitted to me that he does not find her sexy in the slightest. Why? "She sends out 'don't touch, stay away' kinds of messages. She told me that her husband never touched her unless he wanted sex, and she's taken this into her everyday life. She won't let anyone touch her because she still unconsciously feels it's going to lead to sex. And she doesn't touch anyone either."

There are two kinds of touch: accidental and on purpose. In singles bars some women "accidentally" lean forward toward a man while seated next to him, resulting in a brush or breast touch. Julius Fast tells about a woman who was able to use accidental touch to great effect. She would allow her thigh to brush against that of the man she was talking to, or her hand to brush his arm—never the type of touch that would be noticed, but gentle, almost subliminal touching.[8]

On purpose touching, when performed by a skillful flirter, can be a work of art. Sometimes it involves the exchange of objects, such as when a woman and man compare eyeglasses, or hand a pen back and forth. All that is needed is a touch that lingers a few milliseconds longer than necessary. When a man lights a woman's cigarette, she can allow her hands lightly to touch his. Another good way to use touching is to wait until he says something funny. Then, as you are laughing, playfully touch him on the arm or shoulder.

Marilee used touching effectively on a blind date she had with John. "We sat over dinner and dessert for hours, side by side in a booth. It seemed our arms kept brushing, and even our thighs, when I crossed my legs. Pretty soon those accidental touches weren't so accidental. I think I made some comment on the size of his hands, how I liked his hands, and we let our hands touch. We compared hand sizes, the length of our fingers. He took my hand and held it palm up. Pretty soon we were holding hands, and by the end of the night we had both of our hands intertwined. It happened so naturally I really can't pinpoint all of the steps."

Stepping Into a Man's Comfort Zone.   To men, touching is synonymous with sex, and so is physical proximity. A woman who pulls backward when a man dances with her, for instance, who holds herself away and keeps actual physical space between herself and her partner, is communicating that she doesn't want to be close to him. Sexy women show a certain ease about touching, as if they have relaxed certain barriers within themselves.

"Sexy women are more open," one man pointed out. "Much more apt not to hold back if you put your hand on their shoulder, more apt to stand close in your comfort zone."

Body space—the distance people keep between themselves and others when they are talking to them—is an important element in flirting. If a woman steps into a man's "close personal distance," that is, getting within 1-1/2 to 2-1/2 feet of him, she's signalling interest.[9]

Seated in a bar, a woman can get closer to a man's body space by leaning toward him, a ploy often seen at singles watering holes. People who go regularly to singles clubs soon learn to read the body language of the couples they see talking together. If the couple is standing rather far apart, not leaning toward each other, with one or both gazing around the room, singles correctly interpret this as "not interested," or "just friends." Couples standing closer than 2-1/2 feet who are looking at each other, leaning toward each other, or touching, are correctly interpreted as being paired up for the evening and will be left alone.

Display Gestures.   Smiling, eye contact, and touching are all conscious behaviors, easily available to any woman, but there is a whole class of gestures that are done on an unconscious level. But "unconscious" does not mean ineffective—far from it. And some women know how deliberately to make these gestures. Some of the most powerful signals are "preening," or "display" gestures. A woman touches her body or some object in such a way as to show off the fact that she's interested.

Cynthia Kline gives a class in flirting to men in Seattle, and she tells her male students that if a woman is interested in them, she'll show it by toying with some object she is holding, such as a ring, key ring, or wine glass. She may even touch or stroke some part of herself, such as the back of her neck or her hair.[10]

The messages a woman transmits when she does this are simple and effective: She's saying through primitive body language that she would really like to have the man doing the touching. Another sure, no-mistake sign of sexual sparks flying is when a woman runs her hand up and down her thigh, or over her hips. Such erotic gestures are usually unconscious, says Kline—but they are quite honest.

An article in *New Woman* lists these tell-tale, sexy gestures at length: " . . . a hand to the back of the head, picking a few artfully arranged stray curls up off the nape of your neck; lots of self-touching in the chest area; finger your necklace, your earrings; lick guacamole off a finger, hold your glass up to your mouth. . . ."[11]

Hair gestures are very effective, and have a great deal of sexual meaning in flirtation, contends Desmond Morris. A woman repeatedly plays with her hair as she talks to a man. She runs her fingers through it, brushes it back, toys with it, flips it.

"These unconscious grooming movements indicate that the female is unwittingly saying, 'I want to improve my looks for you.' Without realizing it she is transmitting powerful invitation signals to the male."[12]

"Funny, I do play with my hair a lot when I'm with a man," admitted Rachel, 25. "It's shoulder-length and curly, and I enjoy touching it because it's so soft. But I tend to play with it more when there's a man around. I'll fool around, pushing up the hair at the back so it's almost in a bun or French twist, then I'll let it fall down again. Or I'll just fluff it up a little with my fingers. My boyfriend seems to love it when I do that and he'll reach out and touch me, or tell me how much he likes my hair. I guess I reserve those gestures for when I'm feeling sexy, and it seems to work."

There are any number of effective display signals. One man buttonholed me to tell me a list of signals that a woman uses in a bar or lounge setting to show she's available. "She rubs her hand up and down on the glass she's drinking out of. Or she runs her fingertip around the rim of the glass—that's supposed to be very sexy. Another one is where she rubs her finger around her lips, or pulls or plays with her ear. And of course when she's crossing or uncrossing her legs."

Once in a restaurant the use of a pair of glasses worked almost too well. I was dining by myself in a very nice Chicago hotel, thinking to myself that life "on the road" promoting a book could sometimes be lonely indeed. Across the aisle and down the row of booths, a distinguished-looking man in his 60s was dining alone also. I found my gaze wandering to him, as I wondered if he, too, found it oppressive to eat alone.

I wear glasses, and happen to need bifocals, which I'm too proud to break down and buy. I solve the problem in restaurants by taking off my glasses to eat or read a menu. The print immediately comes into clear focus.

On this particular evening, I took my glasses off to read the menu, and then I took them off several times to see my food, again to read the dessert menu when the waiter brought it. Just as I finished ordering, the man I had been observing suddenly appeared at my table and asked if he could join me. He was well-dressed and on close inspection seemed even more distinguished—so on a whim, I said yes.

While I poked at my strawberry cheesecake, we chatted. I was astonished to learn that he had been drawn to my table by my nearsighted byplay with my glasses. "You kept fooling with your glasses, taking them on and off, and I was intrigued. I wondered what you were doing, I thought you were flirting with me."

Later, back in my room (alone, to the gentleman's discreet disappointment) I thought over the incident and realized that he was probably right. I *had* been unconsciously flirting, and the script went something like this. I noticed the man, wondered about him, and had positive thoughts about him. It was then that I began toying with my glasses, the unconscious thought being, 'I want to take off my glasses for you, I want to look my best for you.'

Other Body Movements.   There are numbers of other body movements that are used in flirtation, says Givens, and one of the most effective is shoulder-moving, when the woman gives a small, delicious shrug, drawing her upper arms closer to the center of her body. Or she gazes over her shoulder, giving the man a slight, inviting smile.

"I use my body; I use my shoulders," one woman explained to me. "I look over my shoulder or move the shoulder. I was a dancer when I was young, and that part of me still comes into play. A dancer looks at herself a lot in the mirror and learns how to pose. If she's trying to appeal, naturally her poses will be more becoming. I sit more with crossed legs, my shoulders in, and I look over my shoulders, revealing just a little bit of 'me,' as opposed to a lot. Like, 'Not everybody can see it,' that kind of thing."

Leaning toward the man is another flirtation device, often seen at club meetings when singles are mingling. Two people are seated or standing near each other, and their bodies lean toward each other almost as if there is some invisible connection between them.

I remember being at a discussion group and seeing one woman sitting on the floor next to an attractive man, who was seated in a chair. The woman didn't seem to notice him, but she kept leaning toward him, sitting so near to him that her shoulders kept "accidentally" brushing his calf. This was also a way of penetrating his comfort zone. After a while she put out her hand and began tracing figures in the plush nap of the carpet. Over and over she toyed with the carpet, tracing a very sensuous oval. Later I saw the two in a close *tête-à-tête* near the refreshment table.

Cocking, tilting, or "tossing" the head is another flirtation gesture, more often used by women than by men. The "forward head tilt" is an effective signal that Givens observed often in his studies. Here the woman tilts her head forward so that she has to raise her eyes to meet the man's gaze. (This is very flirtacious, the exact opposite of the backward head tilt, where the person tips the head *back,* chin in the air, and stares at you through half-slitted eyes, the expression being one of arrogance, superiority, and disdain.)[13]

Flashing rings, or ringless fingers, is one way that women can indicate they find a man alluring. As one man pointed out to me, "The restaurant situation is ideal for flirting. You can have a vignette at 50 feet away, flashing the rings. It's what you do or don't do. The left hand comes up to touch the hair or the eyes. . . . Even if they are wearing a wedding ring, you don't know what to think. Marriage today means very little, and plenty of married women flirt."

In a bar setting, women who are feeling flirty may also do a "solitary dance." That is, while they are seated, they keep rhythm to the beat of the music—a signal to any watching men that they are not only enjoying themselves, but eager to dance.

And leg language, mentioned in Chapter 5, is often used in flirting, where the woman crosses and uncrosses her legs, unconsciously touches her knees or thighs, or sits with the legs apart, which is symbolically open and inviting.

Using the Voice.   Many of the men I interviewed mentioned that a woman's soft voice is important to them, and as anthropologist Givens points out, this may have deep biological significance. Remember, part of the purpose in flirting is for the woman to indicate "submissiveness," to show the male that she won't be aggressive toward him. According to Givens, when a woman's voice is softer and higher pitched, like the voice used to speak to young children or animals, this is much less threatening to the male.

Some women are also skilled at using the voice on two levels. The first level is very "surface" or innocuous, simply whatever she is talking about, but the other part of her voice occurs on a deeper, sexy level. There is a way of injecting smiles and warmth into a voice-tone, a delicately hidden laughter, or perhaps emphasis on a certain word or syllable, or even the unconscious choice of words that could be taken to have a double meaning.

"I often use words with a double meaning at work," Candy told me. "And I don't even mean to—but it does put the conversation on a more sexual level."

Singling the Man Out.   As I talked to men and women, I began to get a sense that there are certain characteristic ways that sexy women signal men that it would be safe to approach them. As one woman told me, "Our society still directs that if the woman doesn't speak first, the man won't speak to her. You have to make an effort, at least say hello, to initiate a conversation."

Singling the man out is a time-honored way of initiating a flirtation—an act that takes a certain amount of confidence, which is one of the main characteristics of sexy women to begin with.

"Sometimes women flirt just by breaking out of the observable, normal routine and doing something they wouldn't do with anyone else, like sitting down beside you to talk to you, or including you in some act or conversation," said Phil, an auto executive. Phil has recently married a woman who he met in just this way—she came up to him at a party and sat down beside him, starting a conversation.

Joycelyn, 36, says, "One of the ways I flirt is by going to a party and looking around to see who are the best-looking men in the room. Then over the course of the party I try to go up to each one and start a conversation with him, or else join the conversation group he's in. It's really easy. You just wait until they say something, then comment on what they just said. I try to say something mildly intriguing. They'll respond with a little bit of surprise and start asking me questions."

Singling out is especially effective, because often the man will not initiate anything, out of reluctance, shyness, or fear of rejection. Last year I had a speaking engagement at a Parents Without Partners chapter in Miami, and one of my women friends accompanied me—a woman I later was able to interview as one of the "sexy women" for this book. Both of us noticed the tall, shy-looking, ruggedly handsome man seated in the row behind us. He hadn't talked to anyone all evening, although he was looking around him interestedly.

Within five seconds after my talk was finished, Joann rose from her seat and made a beeline for the next row. Her face wreathed in friendly smiles, she sat down beside him and started a conversation. A shy man, Del probably never would have approached Joann on his own—but he ended up inviting her for dinner the following night.

Looking Accessible.   Men *are* afraid of rejection, especially if they perceive that the woman is especially attractive or sexy.

All men have undergone experiences something like this: he approaches a pretty woman, smiles, asks her to dance, and she says no. The man backs away, feeling bewildered and a bit angry, thinking something like, 'Couldn't she have accepted one dance with me just to be polite?' After a man has been rejected in this way a few times, he starts learning to look for signs of interest before he tries to get close to anyone else.

Bill, who has only average looks, talked to me bitterly about his experiences with rejection. "I've been burned enough that I don't just go up to any woman anymore. I'll look around for a woman who looks friendly or who has been sitting there for a while and hasn't been asked to dance. I can ask her and I know she'll accept."

Looking accessible is the key. Danielle, in a bar, is often approached by men who want to dance with her. How does she accomplish this? "I catch their eye, hold eye contact a little longer than a person normally would. I smile a little. I wouldn't sit with my arms folded, looking at the floor, or being too involved in something to stop and have a conversation. If you go out to dinner by yourself, don't bring a book with you, but bring a magazine and just flip through it."

Looking accessible is partly a matter of mental attitude. Keep pleasant, *"I'm having fun"* thoughts in your mind, so that they'll create an open, receptive expression on your face. Face outward into the room, don't stare at a table top or the wall. If there is an activity going on, watch the activity with as much sparkling interest as you can muster. Look around, keep your eyes moving, as if you were enjoying the whole scene.

Although it may be more comfortable to sit with your arms folded across your chest, don't. Such a position often signifies that a woman is feeling judgemental, or is not really open to approach.

In a bar-lounge, don't surround yourself with a pack of five or six girlfriends, all of you laughing at your own jokes. Instead, go with only one girlfriend, and sit at the bar or an area near the bar, where there is a great deal of circulation going on. Talk vivaciously with your friend, but keep looking around the room, catching the eye of someone who interests you.

At a party, looking accessible means being on your feet and circulating, rather than plopping yourself in a chair in the living room where only a few people can talk to you. At a dance, it means walking around as much as possible, looking around the room, circulating, talking to others, smiling, looking as if you are having fun.

Find Something to Compliment.   Most of the sexy women I talked to said that one of their favorite ways to flirt is to find something about the man to compliment. This works extremely effectively to show interest and to intrigue the man.

"A woman complimenting me on my physical looks or other achievements gives me what you'd call 'a big head,'" said one good-looking 31-year-old sales manager. "I like that. Sometimes it's hard to distinguish whether the compliments are sincere, but I assume they are sincere, and I can be taken in by compliments."

"Compliments feed my ego," admitted another man. "This works in any situation. A woman could find the most attractive part of me—either in my personality or in my dress—and praise that. Don't pick on my long toenails, though!"

Compliments can be very direct. Tracey, in her late 30s, told me about complimenting a man she'd met at a cocktail party. "We were talking on the couch, and somehow the subject got onto physical attractiveness. So I just came right out with it. I said, 'You're very sexually attractive, does that ever make your life more difficult?' It had a question tacked on to it that took some of the pressure off it, and allowed him to go ahead and answer the question, rather than just stammer. But it really worked. He was totally flattered, and we ended up having a relationship."

Another good way to compliment is to single out something in the man that others may not have seen, hitting something that is really *him*. Lila told me about meeting Doug, the man she's living with now, at a divorce workshop.

"The topic was sexuality, and Doug went ahead and told the whole group about this one-night stand he'd had that hurt him very much. He was so honest that I was quite intrigued. I decided that he was a very open man who wore his heart on his sleeve—and I had to meet him. So afterwards I went up and approached him with a compliment. What I said was, 'Your comments made the whole discussion. You took what could have been an embarrassing giggle session and turned it into something meaningful.'

"He was pleased by what I'd said, you could just see him responding all over. We talked for hours, left to have coffee together, and I didn't get home until 4:00 in the morning. Later as I got to know Doug better I learned that he prides himself on his sensitivity, his ability to express his feelings well. As it turned out, if I'd searched for hours, I couldn't have found a better compliment than the one I did give him."

Not Being Dismal or Heavy.   Flirting is by its very nature light-hearted, a happy activity that is totally absorbing to both male and female. When you are flirting, you can't think about problems, or stark, life-is-a-drag realities—and you don't want to. Therefore any talk of dismal or heavy topics is like putting a rock in a soap bubble—it will drop right through and destroy the flirtation.

As Judy, 41, advised me, "When I'm talking to a man I try to focus on the positive, fun aspects of things, not the negatives. I know one woman who is like a broken record about her divorce. I can hardly stand to be around her for more than about ten minutes at a time. One day she came up and asked me why she didn't get dates. I told her to stop talking about her ex. Men don't want to hear all that sad horribleness. Sure, they have to hear your story, but why not wait until you know them better, and even then, don't make it a long drawn-out thing."

Another 26-year-old woman agreed. "How do I turn it on, the flirting? Prolonged eye contact, little jokes, making light of things. Say nothing that is negative, only positive things, it's not really conscious, it's just how I feel."

Sprinkling Conversation with Slightly Risque Jokes or Being Very Open in Talk.   Most sexy women talk or hint about sex, at least "sometimes," universally agreed the men I surveyed. And the women admitted that they do, on occasion, use flirty, half-sexy jokes and remarks.

Said one man, "When sexy women are flirting, they are responsive, not offended by a joke, and you don't see any of that 'get out of here' turn-off. They are open, they laugh, they play along. Sometimes the humor can be suggestive, but that's later on, first off it is just teasing. I came from a big family and I grew up teasing, so when I flirt, I tease. If she teases back, that's very flirtacious to me. Later it can turn more sexual but not at first. But if the suggestiveness is instigated from the other side, I find that attractive."

"I talk very openly and honestly," says Sue. "I just say the same kind of things I would say to a very good friend, sometimes sexual in nature, if that's the way the talk runs, and I'm not afraid to discuss sex with a man."

Adds Jenny, "When I flirt I smile a lot, I laugh at what they say. It helps if you're a bit witty, if you can come back with a joke just a little risque without being obscene. But if you go overboard they think it's serious."

Thinking of Something to Talk to the Man About.   Believe it or not, many men need help in holding up a flirtation. As soon as the by-play starts, a man begins getting uneasy feelings: *She's attractive, but does she like me? Is it an accident she was looking at me like that? If I talk to her will she reject me? Should I show interest in her, and if so, when? Should I ask to buy her a drink?*

When women don't flirt, a man has to carry the conversation and think of things to say. One man told me that he isn't good at that. "If a man is slightly nervous, he'll be relieved if the woman can ask enough questions to get the conversation going. And the very fact that she does, shows that she's interested in him. Sexy women will give you something to talk about with them. 'Here's what I do, I'm inviting you to talk to me about it.' She isn't making small talk, and yet she is; that's the basis of any small flirtation I've ever done," said one attorney.

Asking Small Favors.   There is a book in circulation targeted at men, entitled *How To Pick Up Girls.* Word in publishing circles is that the book did tremendously well, but that its companion volume, *How To Pick Up Men,* did poorly, because women don't like to think of themselves as "picking up" anyone.

But when a woman asks a favor of a man, the connotations of "picking him up" are erased. The contact saves face for both: After all, she did ask the favor, and the whole transaction can take place on that level. But the man is also being given the chance to pursue further if he wishes.

One woman I talked to attends many singles parties held in private homes, to which she totes her own bottle of wine. Her first act on arriving at the party is to go to the kitchen with her wine, and ask a man where the corkscrew is. Then she begs a favor: Will he help her get the cork off? Many of these contacts start a flirtation going.

I gave Wendy, 25, a stack of male questionnaires for my book and asked for her help in getting men to interview. Wendy took the surveys to work. Two days later I received a gleeful phone call: "Those questionnaires were *great,* Julie! They worked like a charm. I got to walk up to every good-looking man in the entire building . . . and two of them asked me out." Having a small favor to ask of these men gave Wendy a good excuse for approaching, and the men could either accept the transaction on that level, or flirt further.

Sharing Food or Other Items.   Sharing can be extremely intimate, and is a warm way of flirting often used by sexy women. Sharing one's bottle of wine, offering a man a taste of your drink, or a bite of your submarine sandwich . . . these are all potentially very sexy signals. We don't share with strangers, and any act that involves the sharing of food is especially significant.

Several years ago I attended a reunion of the Bureau of Social Aid in Ann Arbor, where I had worked as a young social worker. One of the men came up to me and started to reminisce about an incident I had completely forgotten. It was about a sandwich. "I remember it so clearly," he told me. "It was bologna and lettuce with little bits of hard butter on the bread . . . and you shared with me. You *shared.*"

Gail told me about a flirty technique she sometimes uses on a dinner date. "I order dessert at the end of the meal—something very rich and sinful, like a fancy torte or mud pie, something showy. Then I suggest that the man split it with me. Most of them really get into it, finding it very seductive, especially if we eat off the same plate. I remember I did this with one guy, and we happened to order a strawberry ice cream pie. The pie was pink, even the color was sexually suggestive. He made several veiled remarks about that as we slowly ate the pie. Wow, it turned out to be like something from *Tom Jones*. I couldn't believe how turned on he got, the whole thing was just incredible."

Once, on a golf weekend I attended, one of the men complained that he wanted to go swimming in the hotel pool with the others, but had forgotten his bathing suit. I happened to have a pair of shorts with me that had an elastic waist, and I offered to loan those shorts to Ed.

He did have narrow hips, and managed to get them on. He wore them to swim both days, and returned them to me the following week, and ever since then there has been a special bond between us because I'd loaned him something so personal, and, as he put it, "saved my weekend."

Dance Flirting.   Dancing with a man is a powerful opportunity to transmit sexuality, as most sexy women instinctively know. One man talked to me about women he meets at dances: "Sexy women have attributes that make you want to be close. You can tell when you're dancing with a woman like that and be correct 90 percent of the time. One woman I was dancing with took my hand and enfolded it on the upper part of her chest, she actually pulled me toward her and made my stiffness go away. She let me know that she enjoyed being close and wanted me to touch. She made moves, and took the tenseness away from that first meeting and touching. Being the warm and cuddly type is so important."

Women who go to dances should be aware that most women fast-dance with a man in a perfunctory manner, as if he was just anybody. They look around the room, eye others on the dance floor, or even ignore their partner. The man picks up on it—"hey, we're just dancing." No chemistry is transmitted, or very little.

To turn the power way *on,* all you need to do is reverse that. Dance with the man as if he is your partner, and focus all your attention on him. Look him in the eyes, not all the time but occasionally, and turn when he does so that you are facing him, not looking aside. Pick up on some steps of his, so that it looks as if you are really a pair.

Do little hip-wiggling things, smile, lean forward to talk to him in the middle of the music, or brush against him and take his hand for a couple of seconds. In other words, let him know that you are dancing with *him,* that he is special.

However, when the slow, dreamy music comes on, then you change your techniques slightly. When your body is pressed against his, you need to be careful about coming on too suggestively, as it's not unheard of for a man to get an erection on the dance floor. Yet you must relax enough so that he senses you are physically at ease with him. One good way to do this is to follow his movements expertly, moving your body in an exact mirror replica of his. Even poor dancers have told me, in astonishment, that I make them feel like good dancers because I follow *exactly,* using the movements of his chest and abdomen as my cues.

Other slow-dance cues you can give a man include folding his hand close to your shoulder, wrapping your arms around his neck, or dancing cheek to cheek. When the fast music starts up again, act a little reluctant to move out of his arms. This transmits a powerful message, too.

Ginnie agreed. "Dancing close, maybe cheek to cheek, is very sexy and puts the man at ease. But you don't have to be sluttish about it, you don't have to come on strong with a lot of hip-grinding or anything, you can be very ladylike and still intrigue the hell out of him."

Lots of flirting does go on out on the dance floor. "I can be outrageous, and when I'm dancing some of my body movements are on purpose," admits Corinne, a lush 40-year-old blonde. "I love to flirt to *Jump,* by the Pointer Sisters. Another time I was dancing with a man and they played that one by Kenny Rogers, *'Why Don't You Stay,* and . . . well, we left."

What about getting downright sexy and funky? Most women reserve this behavior for someone they already know and feel comfortable with. Ginnie told me that if she's with someone she's already being sexual with, and she just wants to have some good, seductive fun on the dance floor, she becomes much more bold.

"First, I only dance real sexy at a disco someplace where no one knows me anyway. That makes me feel freer. This works best when you're wearing a full skirt. Just move over slightly from the conventional dance position so that you're facing him belly button to belly button. Now, in rhythm to the music, grind your pelvis into his—very slowly, very subtly, so that he knows you're doing it but no one else on the dance floor does. Undulate yourself a little. The full skirt will hide most of it, and no one else will really notice. This will drive him crazy, believe me."

Axioms of Sex Appeal

1. The first thing that happens in flirting, on an instinctive, biological level, is that the man must satisfy himself that his partner is not going to be physically aggressive. Certain submissive behaviors do assure the man that it's safe to approach a woman. Aggressive body language, on the other hand, may be a sexual turn-off.

2. A woman can send out seductive body messages even though she doesn't intend to. Such messages include long periods of smiling, looking into the man's eyes and then averting the eyes, speaking in a soft, high voice, stretching, smiling, and preening the hair.

3. Smiling is a vital part of flirting. "A maid that laughs is half taken."

4. Eye contact is extremely important to flirting also, and takes many forms—the room-encompassing look, the sidelong look, the up-and-down look, the riveting look, and prolonged eye contact.

5. Touching is another strong signal, used by sexy women to maximum effect. This can be touching the man's arm to emphasize a point, or touching him while exchanging objects such as pens or glasses. It can also be "accidental" touch, such as when a woman's thigh brushes against a man's.

6. Stepping into a man's body space or comfort zone is another way to increase the voltage of contact with a man. Women in singles bars frequently lean closer to a man, indicating their strong interest.

7. Display or preening gestures, such as fluffing up the hair, adjusting a necklace, playing with a glass or some other object you are holding, licking guacamole off a finger, all show sexual interest. These are unconscious messages saying, 'I would like my body to look good for you.'

8. Other body movements can be effective, too. These include using the shoulders, cocking or tilting the head, flashing your ring fin-

ger, crossing or uncrossing the legs, or doing a little "dance in place" to the rhythm of music.

9. A woman's voice is important in flirtation, for when it is soft, it lets a man know she will not be aggressive or rejecting. If a voice has a warm, "smiling" quality to it, men will tend to find it very attractive.

10. Singling the man out—cutting him out of a crowded room by starting a conversation or sitting down with him—is an extremely effective way to begin a flirtation.

11. Looking accessible is very important in terms of body language. This is because most men have been rejected often enough to be wary, and many tend to hang back until the woman has shown some signs of interest first. Ways to look accessible include sitting facing the room, allowing your eyes to rove around the room, keeping a happy expression on your face, not looking down or crossing the arms.

12. Never be dismal or heavy if you want to start a flirtation—any talk of depressing topics is like putting a rock in a soap bubble. It will drop right through and destroy the flirtation.

13. Sprinkle your conversation with a judicious selection of slightly risque jokes, or be open in your talk. Most sexy women do talk or hint about sex, at least sometimes, according to the men I surveyed.

14. Other effective moves that women have made include helping the man to carry the conversation, asking small favors of him to give him a chance to flirt, sharing food or other personal items.

15. When dancing with a man you want to attract, don't be perfunctory, gazing all around the room, but rather act as if *he* is your partner and focus all your attention on him. Smile, lean forward to talk to him or touch him, look him in the eyes. When slow dancing, let your body relax, dance close, follow him very closely, and act reluctant to leave his arms when the music is over.

7

Enhancement Factors

I like a woman who's a challenge.
She's not playing hard to get—
she is hard to get.

—Male interviewee

Some women show noticeable changes in appearance as soon as a man appears on the scene. I was interviewing Kelly in a bar-lounge when suddenly a man she knew appeared, calling a greeting to her. Animatedly she waved to him, her face undergoing an instant transformation. Before, talking to me, she had been fairly serious, earnest. Suddenly she sparkled. It was almost as if a light had ignited inside her, turning her from modestly attractive, to very pretty indeed.

Patricia, another woman I interviewed, is much the same way. She, at 32, shows two sides to others. Around women she is gossipy, frank, letting her face fall into its natural expressions. But around men there is a second Pat, bubbly, gay, teasing, super-vivacious. Her face lights up with animation, her eyes almost wicked in their sparkle.

It's true that men and women do undergo certain body changes as they prepare for a sexual encounter. Their bodies sag less, they stand up straighter, more erect and alert. Their eyes brighten, their smiles are more sparkling.

Sex appeal is a complex mechanism, and there are many things that enhance it—built-in factors that have to do with behavior and situation. I call these "enhancing" factors, and women should know that these factors do exist, and how to use them.

For instance, there is a myth perpetuated among high-school age boys that girls with large breasts are sexier, more available, and like sex more. Girls with large breasts suffer embarrassments, catcalls in hallways, whistles on the street.

"Boys often read large breasts as a sign of sexual readiness and some women tell us they actually got the reputation of being "fast" simply on the basis of their anatomy," say Lorna J. Sarrell and Philip M. Sarrell, in their book, *Sexual Turning Points: The Seven Stages of Adult Sexuality*.[1]

And feminist Susan Brownmiller adds, "The assumption of a ready-to-go nature in big-breasted women is reminiscent of the time when generous sexuality was assigned to large, meaty thighs, and the phrase, "She has no thighs," implied an erotic stinginess."[2]

What this means is that women endowed with C cup—or larger—breasts have one automatic extra going for them. In the minds of some men, they are sexier—simply because of the situation; they happen to have large breasts. They do not have to do anything; their anatomy does it for them.

This, then, is one enhancing factor: *Large breasts are considered by some men to be automatically indicative of sexiness.* Fair or not, that's the way it is, and if you have well-endowed bosoms, you might as well relax and take advantage of the gifts mother nature bestowed on you.

But there are other enhancing factors more available to all of us, regardless of our bra size.

The Selectively Hard-to-Get Phenomenon.   I can remember my grandmother, who must have been born in 1882, earnestly telling me that if I played "hard to get" with the boys, I would have better luck. As our mothers or grandmothers insisted, does it really enhance a woman's desirability if she plays "hard to get"? Researchers at the University of Wisconsin delved into this frustratingly complex question, at first with a great deal of difficulty.

Elaine Walster and her associates tried several experiments, with college students and even with prostitutes, but found themselves frustrated and about to give up. All they had learned was that hard-to-get women presented certain problems to men. They were *too* hard to get, making the men feel tense.

"Since she was not particularly enthusiastic about you, she might stand you up or humiliate you in front of your friends. She was likely to be unfriendly, cold, and to possess inflexible standards," Walster wrote in the *Journal of Personality and Social Psychology.*[3]

Not a date guaranteed to be fun.

What about the easy-to-get woman, then, the one who accepts dates too eagerly? Dating her might be relaxing, and an ego-booster, but the men reported disadvantages here too.

"Such a woman might be easy to get, but hard to get rid of. She might 'get serious.' Perhaps she would be so oversexed or over-affectionate in public that she would embarrass you. Your buddies might snicker when they saw you together. After all, they would know perfectly well why you were dating *her*."

Apparently an easy-to-get woman wasn't a very desirable date either.

Then who was? Finally the secret dawned on the research group. There are really two important determinants on how much a man likes a woman. One is how hard or easy she is for him to get. The other is how hard or easy she is for *other men* to get.

Finally they formed a hypothesis: *If a woman has a reputation for being hard to get, but for some reason she is easy for the subject to get, she should be maximally appealing.*

The research group then recruited 71 male summer students at the University of Wisconsin, getting them to join a "computer dating center." When each male arrived to select his "date," he was presented with folders containing information on five women—the same five women each time. The gimmick was that the folders contained a "date selection form," that the woman had supposedly filled out to evaluate other dates she had been offered.

One of the five women appeared uniformly easy to get—she was enthusiastic about dating all five of the men assigned to her. One woman was very hard to get—she was not enthusiastic about any of her dates, including the subject. Another woman indicated minimum enthusiasm for four of her dates, but extreme enthusiasm for the experimental subject. Two women didn't have any date selection forms in their folder at all.

Then the researchers quizzed the men students on a number of factors about their prospective dates, from how friendly-unfriendly they were, to their overall liking of the woman. The woman who was picky about other men, but liked the male subject, won hands down.

"When we examine the men's choices in dates, we see that the selective woman is far more popular than any of her rivals," wrote Walster. "Nearly all subjects preferred to date the selective woman. When we compare the frequency with which her four rivals (combined) are chosen, we see that the selective woman does get far more than her share of dates."

The researchers reached a further, interesting conclusion, "It appears that a woman can enhance her desirability if she acquires a reputation for being hard to get, and then, by her behavior, makes it clear to a selected romantic partner that she is interested in him."[4]

Some of the men I interviewed concurred with this conclusion, saying things like, "A man doesn't want to think that a woman is being that way (practicing sexy behavior) for all men, but he wants it to be just for him."

The Gain Phenomenon. The "gain phenomenon" is another enhancement factor, and simply put, it means that *people are more attracted to a person who is initially punishing and then rewarding, than to one who is always rewarding.*

A University of Illinois study made video tapes of actresses carrying on conversations. In some of the tapes, the woman acted "coldly" throughout the interview, in another tape she was entirely warm, in others she was first cold, then warm. Subjects were then asked how much they thought the man would be attracted to the woman in each instance.

What were the results? "When the stimulus female was first cold, and then warm, the subjects believed that the man would like her more, and be more likely to want to see her again," concluded the researchers.[5]

Men have another word to describe this phenomenon, and that is selective, or challenging. A selective woman might be a little cold at first but she then warms up to the man, indicating that she prefers *him,* to other men. Men are universally flattered when they think a woman has rejected others in favor of them.

The High-Anxiety Factor. Another fascinating aspect of sexuality that researchers have discovered is the "high-anxiety factor." What it means is that sexual attraction or sexy feelings occur more often under conditions of high emotion, such as anger, fear, or pain.

Various studies have been undertaken to prove this. In one Canadian study, a classroom of college students was deliberately and viciously berated over test scores, in order to anger them. This group and a control group were then given brief stories to write, in which sexual content would be measured. The group that scored highest on sexy thoughts was the class that had been stimulated by anger.[6]

In another Canadian study, 85 men were tested as to how they would react to an attractive woman under conditions of danger. The setting for the experiment was two bridges over the Capilano River in North Vancouver, British Columbia. One of the bridges was a scary one—it was a five-foot-wide suspension bridge, with very low handrails that overlooked a 230 foot drop to rocks and rapids below. This structure had an alarming tendency to tilt, wobble, and sway. The other bridge was a prosaic, solid, wooden structure over a small, shallow rivulet that ran into the main river.

As these men crossed the bridges, they were approached by a female interviewer, who said she was doing a project for her psychology class, and asked them to write a short story based on a TAT picture (Thematic Apperception Test). She gave the men her phone number and told them they could call her if they had any further questions. Then the same procedure was repeated, this time using a male interviewer.

Results? On the anxiety-producing suspension bridge, the stories the men told were significantly higher in sexual content. Half of those who accepted the woman's phone number actually called her back, as opposed to only 2 of 16 who had been on the safe bridge. Almost none of the men telephoned the man who had interviewed them.[7] In other words, conditions of danger made the woman seem sexier!

Another study involved male college students who were left in a room with an attractive female after being told they were both going to get high electrical shocks as part of an "experiment." After the nervousness of anticipation had had a chance to work on them, the men were questioned about the woman with whom they'd been in the room. How much would they like to ask her for a date? How much would they like to kiss her?

Other groups were told they would get low shocks, or were put in a room with a male confederate. What happened? Feelings of sexual attraction were *higher* among the students who'd been told that both they and the woman would get high shocks. ". . . strong emotion per se increases the subject's sexual attraction to the female confederate," concluded the researchers.[8]

"Almost any form of arousal seems to be conducive to love," writes sex researcher H. J. Eysenck in his book, *The Psychology of Sex.* "It does not seem to matter whether it is positive in nature (e.g. excitement or success arising out of amateur dramatics, mountain climbing, or passing an examination), or unpleasant (e.g. danger, fear, pain), though it helps if the experience is shared."[9]

Therefore the conclusion seems clear: A woman who wants to use the "high-anxiety" factor to her own, sexy advantage, simply has to put herself in a spot where men and women experience either high emotions or a certain amount of physical danger. That very danger will enhance her sex appeal, along with the man's sexual thoughts in general. It's no accident that singles groups that sponsor white-water rafting trips, mule trips down canyons, canoe trips, etc., also spawn a number of romances. Danger—even mild risk—sparks sexiness.

What is Beautiful is Good. Another enhancement factor works to the advantage of the physically attractive. Repeated studies have shown that most people automatically assume that attractive people possess more desirable characteristics. Attractive people are viewed as being happier, more sensitive, more sociable, and having better character than their less attractive counterparts, psychologists say, and this has proven true over and over in tests.

Moreover, this assumption that "beauty is good" goes all the way down the ladder to nursery school. One study done in a nursery school showed that adult test subjects *assumed* that a pretty little girl who committed a minor naughtiness (like pulling a dog's tail) did it out of high spirits and was basically well-adjusted. But if a plain little girl did the same prank, the subjects assumed that she would cause further trouble and be maladjusted.[10] Even preschoolers themselves think that a "pretty" or "handsome" child is less likely to be bad.

So a woman who is attractive, or who can transmit the illusion of being attractive, stands a better chance of being considered sexy—along with a lot of other positive traits.

The Closing-Time Factor.   There's a country-western song written by Baker Knight and sung by Mickey Gilley with a title that expresses this enhancement factor in a nutshell: *"Don't the Girls All Get Prettier At Closing Time."* This is the idea that individuals of the opposite sex become more attractive as the time for interacting with them runs short.

Researchers actually used this song as a suggestion, and went out and investigated three bars near the University of Virginia campus. They approached bar patrons who were not talking with a member of the opposite sex, and were not intoxicated, and asked if they would mind answering a couple of questions for a psychological study. How would they rate the members of the opposite sex in the bar for attractiveness on a scale of 1 to 10? This was done at three times in the evening: 9 PM, 10:30 PM, and midnight (closing time was 12:30 AM).

Analysis of the ratings confirmed Gilley's song. The women in the bar *were* seen as prettier as closing time approached. Ratings of the women dipped on the second survey, at 10:30 PM (were the men getting discouraged?), then soared again at midnight when the bars were closing and the time for pickups was running out.

Psychologist James W. Pennebaker concluded that his findings illustrated the theory that, "if you feel your freedom to choose or act is being threatened, you react by liking the threatened option or options more than before."[11]

The Invigorating Effects of Novelty.   Sometimes (sadly for the happiness of some long-term marriages) the *newness* of a partner makes for greater sex appeal to men. Animal behaviorists have learned that male rhesus monkeys show a clear increased interest in sexual activity when new females in the troop go into estrus. Male monkeys caged with the same female for a long time need long periods of foreplay before they can ejaculate. But if the females of two pairs are swapped—in other words, if the males get a new partner—the males can mount and ejaculate without delay.

Is the same true for humans as well? Some evidence indicates that it may be. In one South Seas society, the men bitterly lamented the outlawing of concubinage, insisting that it made them old before their time! And, according to Frank Beach, a sexual researcher, men of our society often do report dramatic increases in sexual ability when they change partners. This may explain some cases of midlife crisis in men, as well as the fact that three-fourths of the husbands studied by Kinsey admitted at least an occasional desire for extramarital intercourse.[12]

So if you are new to a man, untried by him sexually, this alone may enhance your appeal to him.

The "Hang Around Beauty" Effect.   When you're planning to cruise the singles bars, which girlfriend should you choose to accompany you? If you're only average-looking, you're better off when you hang around with good-looking girlfriends, rather than homely-looking ones, researchers have found.

At the University of California at Los Angeles, researchers showed yearbook photos of high school women to a group of male and female undergraduates. The pictures were presented three at a time, with the average-looking woman flanked by various combinations of very attractive, average looking, or unattractive students.

The scientists found that the attractive women exerted a lot of influence. The ordinary-looking women were rated as prettier when their pictures were next to a "fox," than when they were next to another average or plain-looking woman.[13]

"I have a girlfriend who is a knockout blonde," said Marilee. "Men are always drawn to her. She has been calling me and begging me to go out with her and at first I didn't want to do it. I'm more average in looks. I figured all the men would be after her and they'd ignore me. Well, it hasn't turned out that way at all. Actually, when we are together we both attract attention, and a lot of the men who are drawn to us because of her looks end up talking to me and seeming to enjoy themselves. I would say that it isn't a detriment to go out with an attractive friend at all."

Axioms of Sex Appeal

1. Men and women do undergo bodily changes as they ready themselves for interaction with the opposite sex, and many sexy women show noticeable changes in appearance as soon as an attractive man appears on the scene.

2. There are certain myths circulated among young boys, and one of them is that girls with large breasts are sexier, and more "ready to go." This is what I call an enhancement factor—a circumstance that works to build up sex appeal.

3. When a woman plays selectively hard to get—that is, when she is hard for most men to get, but easy for a target man to date—this enhances her desirability the most. If a woman plays hard to get for all men, men may fear she'll be cold or rejecting. If she is *too* easy to get she isn't a desirable date either—men fear she might grow too serious, or be too hard to get rid of.

4. People are more attracted to a person who is initially punishing and then rewarding than to a person who is always rewarding. In one study, the woman men found most attractive on a video tape was the one who first acted cold, then warmed up later.

5. Higher feelings of sexiness or attraction often occur under conditions of anxiety, fear, pain, or physical danger. It is easy to get a man attracted to you sexually if the two of you can interact under conditions of emotional or physical challenge, such as white-water rafting or kayaking.

6. If you are physically beautiful, people automatically assume that you possess other desirable characteristics—in other words, beauty is assumed to be "good."

7. There is a phenomenon called the "closing time factor," based on the country-western song, *"Don't the Girls All Get Prettier At Closing Time."* What it means is that individuals of the opposite sex seem more desirable as the time for interacting with them runs short.

8. Male monkeys experience sexual rejuvenation when they interact with a new partner, and human males may also find novelty in a partner extremely stimulating. In fact, if you are new to a man, this alone may increase your sexiness to him.

9. Average-looking women seem more attractive when they hang out with more attractive ones, studies have found. Pictures of ordinary-looking women were rated as more attractive when they were placed next to those of a "fox." Therefore when choosing girlfriends with whom to tour the local singles lounges, it may be more effective to choose one who is better looking than you are.

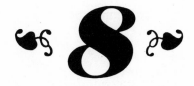

Sexy Women
and Sex

*The allurement that women hold out
to men is precisely the allurement
that Cape Hatteras holds out to sailors: they are enormously dangerous
and hence enormously fascinating.*

—H. L. Mencken,
A Mencken Chrestomathy.

If much of sexiness is in the mind, then *sex* has to be on the minds of sexy women as well. Men certainly believe that it is. They told me over and over that they think that a sexy woman looks as if she likes sex more than the average woman does.

One woman gave me a forthright definition of sex appeal. "Mostly it has to do with whether or not a woman looks as if she'd enjoy a good roll in the hay without taking it all too terribly seriously. Women who are too neat and tidy, who don't look as if they could be mussed up, aren't likely to be much fun in bed. It has to do with a sense of enjoyment of sex and the ability not to talk about it too much. As my long-deceased mother-in-law used to say (always in French), 'Suggestion is a lot more provocative than expression.' "

One of my male friends, 37, good-looking and divorced, is an observer of the human scene, and likes to look for signs of sexuality in women. He feels that he is very good at spotting these small signals. "In my memory there are two women who really showed strong sexy body language. One was years ago. She wasn't particularly well-dressed, but her facial expressions were sexy, the way she moved her body, very uninhibited. It wasn't out of order or anything, but there was something so strong about the way she moved and the way she held her face. I could tell she thinks about sex. And the other one I saw sitting in church. She was a good-looking woman who was playing with her mouth in church, kind of rubbing her fingers around her lips. It was a real strong sign that she was very sensual."

Apparently very-sexy women are at ease with sex, and like it more than the average woman does. They think about it more and often make dates with their husbands—if married—for sex. When sexy women talk with a man at a party, more than half have sexual thoughts about him—at least sometimes.

"I've wondered about other women, if they have the same thoughts I do," confided one woman. "I am very sexually aware. I've read that you never have males and females together unless they are interacting sexually. It's either, yuccch, I wouldn't want that, or how good it would be. At one time I was bothered by that, I pushed thoughts like that aside. Now, yes, I think sexually about a man I am talking to. I think about sex a lot."

"When I see a good-looking man at a party I do look him over sexually," agreed Nita, 30. "It's not so much a conscious thing, but I am very aware of certain parts of that man—his arms, thighs, his tight flat stomach or his buttocks, etc. Sometimes I undress men in my mind. I am interested in imagining what they would look like unclothed. And if I'm having a conversation with a man I do get these flashes of what he'd be like—I can't help it. Not all men, though. Just certain ones."

As some women pointed out, they occasionally get mixed thoughts when meeting a man. As one expressed it, "Sometimes it's contradictory. I meet an attractive man and think about him sexually—then I shy away from him because he's too attractive."

Sexy women like to make love more often. The sexy wives in the *Ladies Home Journal* survey made love three or more times a week, compared to the least satisfied women surveyed, who reported making love once a week or less. The majority of the women I surveyed also preferred making love 3 to 4 times weekly; however, five women said they preferred to have sexual intercourse more than once a day!

LHJ's sexy wives, in fact, love to make love at hours other than bedtime. More than three-quarters said they would make love early in the evening, for example, as compared to only 23 percent of the dissatisfied wives, and 62 percent of all the women the magazine studied. And 95 percent of these women said that when they make love, they don't think about *anything else*.[1]

Male instincts are right—sexy women do enjoy sex. Of the 60 women I surveyed, two-thirds said they "love sex with their partner and greatly look forward to it." A third more said they "enjoy sex with him most of the time." And many said they wished their partner wanted more sex than he does.

But when *Redbook* surveyed its readers, only 32.8 percent said the sexual aspect of their marriage was "very good," and 34.2 percent said it was good—a sharp contrast.[2] Even more interesting is a *Psychology Today* sex survey, which polled a slightly younger group, mostly under age 35. Only 27 percent of these young women rated their sex lives as "very satisfactory"![3]

Just as men fantasize, sexy women also are more orgasmic than ordinary women. More than three-quarters of the sexy *LHJ* wives said they rarely had difficulty climaxing, compared to 72 percent of the unhappy wives who said they did have trouble. The women I surveyed showed similar happy characteristics: About three-quarters said they climax all of the time or most of the time.

Being orgasmic has a positive influence on the way a woman feels about herself sexually, and probably does contribute to sex appeal. Studies have shown that there are some differences in women who are orgasmic as opposed to those who are not. Orgasmic women, for instance, value their sexuality for its own sake, and seek actively to satisfy themselves, focusing on the sexual interaction itself. In other words, they take responsibility for their own climaxes. They are little disturbed by outside noises, believe themselves to be uninhibited, and generally believe that all sexual positions are about equal.

Unmarried college women who have orgasms, according to H. J. Eysenck, are less likely to have conflict with their parents, especially their fathers, and rate themselves freer of sexual inhibitions. They become more aroused from petting, and are more satisfied with their capacity for sexual arousal. They feel that their sex drives are about equal with their partners', and they are more likely to initiate sexual activity.[4]

On the other hand, women who don't climax (and according to Masters and Johnson, between 7 and 10 percent of American women fit this category), tend to focus more on the total ambiance of the situation, such as setting, timing, soft music, closeness, warmth, and sharing. They are not nearly as much aroused by the sex act, enjoy the act much less, are less likely to want a continuation of sexual activity after coitus, are much disturbed by outside noises, and prefer the "missionary" position when making love.[5]

Marilyn Monroe was one of the 7 to 10 percent of women who have never had an orgasm. One of her lovers said that she thought sex got you closer, made you a closer friend.[6]

Do sexy women fake orgasms? Apparently not often. Dr. Joyce Brothers wrote that she once took an informal survey of 40 women she knew to find out how many of them faked orgasms. All of the 40 said that they did about half the time. They explained that they did it so they wouldn't hurt the man's feelings, or because he felt that if she didn't have an orgasm he was a failure as a man.[7] In contrast, of the 60 women I polled, 39 said they *never* fake orgasms, 12 said they do it occasionally, and only 1 said she fakes most of the time.

"Faking an orgasm is like telling a lie," said one woman. "Besides, if you fake he thinks he's pleased you, and you're just teaching him to do all the wrong things."

Another told me rather bitterly that she used to fake orgasms when she was married, "wondering what it was that I was faking. I knew I was supposed to be making a noise about now, so I did." Happily, this woman told me that since her divorce she has stopped faking, and now new self-confidence has spilled over into her sex life—not only does she not have to fake orgasms, she is multi-orgasmic.

Sexy women probably are much better able to talk about what they want and need in bed than ordinary women. Two-thirds of the sexy women I surveyed said they feel comfortable talking to their partner about what they need sexually. In contrast, one survey, done by *Redbook* magazine, found that of the more average readers they surveyed, less than half felt comfortable talking about intimate sexual feelings and desires with their partner.[8]

Ninety-five percent of *Ladies Home Journal's* sexy wives talk during lovemaking (compared to less than half of the least sexy women), and 43 percent tell their husbands what they would like when they are making love. Ninety percent express pleasure (and what greater aphrodisiac could there be for a man than that?)[9]

Sexy women probably tend to be more liberal in accepting the broad spectrum of sexual acts such as cunnilingus and fellatio. In response to my statement, *"There are things my partner wants to try that I feel uncomfortable doing and would prefer not to do,"* three-fourths of the women I surveyed responded either "seldom" or "never." In other words, these sexy women felt comfortable with most aspects of sex, even liberal ones. The *Ladies Home Journal* sexy wives were even more liberal in their eager responses. Almost 90 percent reported that they enjoyed the sexual experiments that their husbands suggested![10]

Repeated surveys have shown that the act men most long for women to perform in bed is oral-genital sex (fellatio). Only 40 percent of the more average *Redbook* readers performed fellatio on their husbands often, with another 44 percent doing this occasionally. And only 34 percent of those who did perform this act described it as very enjoyable, with 38 percent saying they found it somewhat enjoyable.[11]

How often do sexy women initiate sex? Half of the women I surveyed said they suggest or initiate sex 50 percent of the time or more. In fact, one woman said she initiated it with her partner 90 percent of the time, and another woman put her percentage at 95. In contrast, only 43 percent of *Redbook's* readers initiated sex half the time.

However, the sexy women I talked to did match the readers of *Redbook* in one way—the method they used to tell their partner they wanted sex. Figures tallied pretty much down the line, leading me to conclude that most women—sexy or not—let men know when they want sex in just about the same way. More than half (54 percent) caress or cuddle their partners; 31.9 percent tell him directly; 37.8 touch his genitals; 13.6 percent flirt, and 18 percent say "he just knows."

Are sexy women *better* in bed than the average woman? Two-thirds of the men I polled believed that they are, although many men pointed out that exceptionally beautiful women are often less skilled than their plainer sisters—mainly because life has proved to them that they don't have to make much of an effort to be desired.

As writer Sidney Sheldon once said, "Women who are plain and unsexy-looking can be marvelous (in bed) and beautiful women can be terrible. In my bachelor days I went out with a lot of beautiful movie stars and models, but you can never have much fun in bed with girls like that. They're so concerned about their appearance, their clothes, and think about themselves constantly. They don't want their hair messed up when they go to bed with you. . . ."[12]

If anyone is an authority on sexy women it is Bob Guccione, of *Forum, Penthouse,* and *Viva* fame. He insists that "the type of woman who is good in bed is good regardless of her looks. She usually has much greater personal magnetism than other women, no matter how beautiful they are."[13]

Another man agreed. "You're really talking about two different things, sexually appealing and sexual," he said. "Women who exhibit sexuality through their body language usually *are* sexy in bed. They might not be as attractive, as pretty, but you can see they are the sexy ones, really into it. You can tell the difference right away with warm women who like to touch. They make you feel they want to be with you."

One man stressed the importance of fantasy—his. "Alas, my experience in this area is painfully limited," said a 30-year-old teacher. "But my fantasies are boundless. I certainly imagine that sexy women are better in bed—more experienced, more experimental, less inhibited, capable of greater sexual satisfaction. They claw, scream, thrash about, and are, of course, multi-orgasmic."

Male fantasies about women certainly must have a bearing on the whole issue of sex appeal. After all, it is *because* of men that we feel sexy, and even when we feel sexy for ourselves, that still translates back to the fact that it is *men* who find us desirable.

Mary told me about a date she had with a man who had made it apparent that he was falling in love with her. "I brought him back to my house and we did go to bed together, but it was one of those things—sometimes I'm shy when it's the first time with a man. I'll never forget what he said to me afterwards. He said—and I think he really meant this—'I thought you were going to rip my clothes off me.' He apparently thought I was so sexy that he fantasized I would be totally animalistic in my behavior."

According to one study, 89 percent of men fantasize during sexual intercourse, as opposed to 64 percent of women. Dr. Ken Druck, in revealing "secrets men keep," notes that men learn to keep the fascination they have with the female anatomy locked away in their imagination. They read magazines like *Penthouse* and create sexual fantasies for a variety of reasons.

In the fantasy, a man doesn't have to be an expert lover, he can get as much sex as he wants, and he can safely unleash his forbidden desires and lose his inhibitions.

"His fantasy never refuses him anything—and he comes through for her every time. Inside the protective walls of a man's imagination, sex is safe, simple, and has no limits."[14]

One man told me that he has kept copies of *Penthouse* and *Forum* for years, using them as "sex substitutes" during a sexless marriage breakup and subsequent lonely, single times. "All right, that's what those magazines are for," he told me. "and there are a lot of business men in $400 suits who buy that magazine, too, and do you think they buy them for the articles? No way!"

Men do find the sight of exposed genitals a turn-on. In fact, one sex therapist advises her female patients who are shy about exposing their bodies to men, to remember that men are spending millions of dollars yearly on flesh magazines, in order to view female genitals. Said Bud, 36, "Women don't realize that to men their pussy is very, very erotic, it is the focus, the center of everything, and it's no accident that all those pictures in *Penthouse* focus on that part. I think a pussy is beautiful, it's like a flower, a rose with all those pink petals . . . it's just beautiful."

Some women, very private about their bodies, may be astonished by what another man said: "I like it when I'm walking in the health club, and I see some woman working out, and I catch a glimpse of her pussy hairs peeking out through her shorts. That is very sexy. I remember one time at the beach I just about had a heart attack when I walked by this young girl, she was lying on a blanket in a bikini and there was this string coming out of her bikini. She was just kind of playing with it, twirling it about with her fingers."

Leafing through two years' worth of borrowed issues of *Penthouse,* looking for articles that might have a bearing on this book, I was struck by the succession of feelings that surged through me. First was anger . . . was this what men really wanted? Then came disgust and curiosity. But finally the curiosity faded into something else, growing stronger as I turned page after page of glossy, explicit photos.

It began to sink in that whether I liked it or not, these

poses were what men considered bedroom seductive. I began looking at the pictures with new eyes. In many of the photos the woman touched herself or toyed with herself, her lips pouty as if daring the man to approach her. In others, she displayed herself with a frankly lusty come-hither air. There were eye-looks that were boldly sultry, the epitome of "bedroom eyes," repeated again and again. Eyes that looked sex-glazed, self absorbed.

Always, in displaying themselves, these women were totally bold and uninhibited, and the attitude conveyed was that there was nothing, *nothing at all,* that they wouldn't do for their man in bed. This, then, is the male fantasy—the serendipitous sexy woman who will do anything, anything. Could any of that frank uninhibited lust be transferred to my own lovemaking with my lover? That total *abandon,* which is really the main theme of all the poses?

Leafing further, my mind inevitably on lovemaking, I came across further clues to male sexuality. A survey done by *Penthouse* as to reader preferences while lovemaking was enlightening. Eighty percent of the men liked "dirty talk" while making love, and these samples of such turn-on language were voted most effective: "You feel so good inside me," "I want your cock inside me so badly," "You do that so well; you really know how to love a woman," and "You have a beautiful penis."[15]

Apparently (just like women) men need positive reinforcement as to their sexiness—a feedback that sexy women know how to provide. As mentioned earlier, the sexy women surveyed by *Ladies Home Journal,* were exceptionally good at talking in bed. One reader said that she regularly assures her husband as to how sexy he is to her, how handsome he is, how good he smells, how wonderful his muscles feel, etc. "He wouldn't know if I never told him so, and I want him to know he still turns me on, after ten years."[16]

"One thing I do in lovemaking," Beth, 37, told me, "is tell my boyfriend just how sexy I find him physically. You would be amazed at how much he loves this. He is a handsome man, and yet he loves being reassured that I find him physically attractive. It's a turn-on for both of us, as one thing leads to another. . . ."

What about female fantasies? Sexy women, I learned, have

both sex fantasies and romantic fantasies—and some have both. Therapist E. Barbara Hariton did extensive research into women's sexual fantasies and concluded that erotic fantasies are common among women—even far-out fantasies—and these are not escape mechanisms, or signs of neuroticism, as some therapists previously had thought, but healthy signs of a well-integrated personality.

She studied 141 women and interviewed 56 of them, learning that 65 percent of the women regularly fantasized during intercourse, while another 28 percent said they had occasional thoughts during intercourse that could be considered as fantasy. The strongest theme in these fantasies was being with another man (60 percent), or being forced into sex by a faceless, ardent male figure (53 percent "sometimes," 15 percent "very often.") One woman imagined herself a harem slave displaying her breasts to an adoring shiek. She would also imagine herself at a drive-in movie being raped by a man whose face was a "blur." Other fantasies included forced sex, sometimes with more than one man at once, with the woman thoroughly enjoying the fact that she could "turn on" males.[17]

Psychoanalysts have argued about whether such fantasies represent signs that women are innately masochistic, or result from society's repression of women. But Abraham Maslow has noted that women who create submission-type fantasies are *high in self esteem,* while women who really are passive, are *least* likely to have such fantasies.

Says Dr. Hariton, "It may be that a confident woman does not let her own fantasies intimidate her, even if they seem less than idealistic. She accepts and trusts her own experiences and has little need to repress or deny them. She permits herself inexplicable images and ideas without feeling any threat to her integrity or sanity."[18]

But more than half of the women I interviewed said they had romantic fantasies, rather than sexual ones. A romance fantasy might be one in which the woman imagines a soft, tender scenario. The man rescues her, talks to her romantically, or performs some super-romantic act. Kerry told me she sometimes imagines that she is trapped in a stuck elevator with a handsome man who resembles Tom Selleck, spending eight to ten hours there with him talking romantically to her and kissing her.

A romantic fantasy is mostly concerned with talk, or perhaps kissing, but does not go farther than that. "Several men have asked me whether I had fantasies and I come up blank," one woman told me. "Actually I think my fantasies are conversational. I have conversations in my mind with men."

Readers of romance novels know that most romances do contain fantasy material of both types—sexy and romantic. However, even the sex is "romantic" in nature, with pages of long, slow build-up, and orgasms described in terms of rushes of feeling, and beautiful explosions, rather than clinical description.

Kathryn Falk, publisher of *Romantic Times,* writes of the skyrocketing success of the steamy brand of category romance lines like Silhouette Desire, Ecstasy, Intimate Moments, Loveswept, and Rapture. "Romance readers don't want to read of the sex act in graphic terms. Without going into repression and guilt, suffice it to say here that you will not find the words *penis, cunnilingus, sodomy,* or any textbook term in a category romance. . . . Many romance writers collect pretty ways of describing anatomical parts, the cliches now being temple of love, creamy thighs, mound of Venus, etc. Many imaginative new terms and one-liners are being created to keep sex pretty. Women also expect their writers to sweep them into an exciting, loving, and breathless encounter with a Prince Charming, but once in his arms, the readers want their own fantasies to take over. . . ."[19]

Actually women who read romance novels may be sexier than those who don't, according to two psychologists, Claire Coles and M. Johanna Shamp, who quizzed 48 women about their romance reading habits. These romance readers made love with their partners nearly *three times* as often as non-readers, and used the sensuous-scene descriptions to heighten their fantasy lives.[20]

Sex, romance, and fantasy are inextricably mingled with the whole concept of sex appeal, creating an interlocking effect. As both men and women fantasize, something magical and electrical begins to grow. Women who think about sex, love sex, and feel sexually appreciated, transmit these thoughts. And when a man senses these things, the woman becomes even *more* sexy to him.

Axioms of Sex Appeal

1. Sexy women tend to be at ease with sex and like it more than the average woman does. They think about it more and make love more often than the average. They rate their sex lives as highly enjoyable, in sharp contrast to women polled in other surveys.

2. Sexy women are more orgasmic than ordinary women—about three-quarters climax all of the time or most of the time. In fact, being orgasmic has a positive influence both on the way a woman feels about herself sexually and the way she reacts to men.

3. Women who men consider sexy are probably more liberal in bed (a fact long suspected by men), and tend to initiate sex at least half the time—in contrast to more ordinary women, only 43 percent of whom initiate sex half the time.

4. Men tend to believe that sexy women are better in bed than the average woman—but they also point out that exceptionally beautiful women do not always perform in bed as well as their plainer sisters.

5. The pages of *Penthouse* can offer women clues as to what men find alluring. The sight of female genitals is a real turn-on for men, and the self-touching poses and come-hither looks depicted in these magazines are illustrations of what males consider bedroom seductive.

6. Men need positive feedback as to *their* sexiness, too, a feedback that sexy women are exceptionally good at providing. Sexy women talk in bed, and tell their men how good-looking and masculine they are. Men like to hear sexually explicit praise about their bodies and their lovemaking abilities.

7. Women generally have two kinds of fantasies—sexual and romantic. Even far-out sexual fantasies don't necessarily show that a woman is passive or emotionally disturbed. On the contrary, women who allow themselves to "flow" with their fantasies generally have high self esteem.

8. More sexy women have romance fantasies, however, than sexual ones. And it has been learned that readers of romance novels tend to be sexier and enjoy sex more than nonreaders.

9

Choices and Signals

"Where should one use perfume?" a young woman asked. "Wherever one wants to be kissed," I said.

—Coco Chanel

We've all had the experience of meeting people and instinctively taking a liking or disliking to them, maybe just on the flimsy basis of what they were wearing. We might be ashamed, but who hasn't been introduced to a woman in a dress so tight it showed her bra bulges or whose hair was hanging limply, and found that we were . . . well, just not responding to her as well as we might?

Walk into any big department store and see the astonishing riches of clothes—casual, baggy, saggy, bright-hued, wild-striped, sedate, plain, tight, punk, preppy, designer. Every time we buy one of these garments, we are making a *choice,* and we are sending out a signal to other people: *this is who I am, and I've chosen this article to show you.* Every time you get dressed in the morning, you send out messages to the world about how good you feel about yourself, how confident you are, how sexy you feel yourself to be.

Clothing is a uniform, points out David Burns in his book, *Intimate Connections.* It conveys a message and allows you to play a particular role. However, some people dress poorly because of a deep fear of dressing attractively or looking sexy or even of being sensual.

Said Jayne Mansfield, "Deep inside every woman there are certain devices designed to attract a man—devices to attract a man's eyes to what he should be attracted to. I've always sensed this—been aware of it, in my dress and the way I walk."[1]

Over and over as I talked to the sexy women for this book, I heard them tell me, "I dress to please *me,* business-wise and socially. I feel very comfortable just being me and not pretending to be someone else or to please a person temporarily." And yet—somehow those clothes they choose for themselves are also pleasing men.

Women who don't feel sexy, don't dress sexy. This is one of the "vibes" that men pick up on, even in the few short seconds it takes to them to eye a woman on the street or in an elevator. Remember Renee, who had her "fat days"? On those inauspicious mornings, Renee got up and put on a tent dress to hide her imagined bulges. That clothing choice sent out a very strong message, *"I feel fat. I feel unattractive. Don't look at me."*

We can go to any shopping mall and see plenty of women in outfits that project unattractiveness. Writes Carolyn See in *The New York Times,* "The women I knew who weren't loved wore their lovelessness like a badge: sweatshirts with geese on them, and bobby socks, or purple smocks to cover their vodka bellies."[2]

On the other hand, don't we all know women whose figures might not be perfect, but who dress as if they were? Who choose knock-out, tasteful clothing and wear it with zest and confidence, giving you a good feeling just to look at them? Those kinds of choices send out messages, too, *"I feel wonderful and I'm confident and happy."* Now, if you were a man, which would you choose to take a second look at?

The message is simple. If clothing choices are messages we are sending to the world, then that gives us the opportunity to send out the kind of messages we *want* to send—upbeat ones, positive ones, sexy ones.

Clothing

What sort of clothes do men really like? For clothing to be successful in sex appeal, it must emphasize the femaleness of a woman, rather than the male. According to Helen Andelin, author of *Fascinating Womanhood,* a woman should avoid "male" type fabrics and styles, or if she does wear them, they should be softened by a feminine style, color, or trim. "Otherwise," said Andelin, "They can give no help in making men realize how unmanlike—how womanly—you are! They cannot strive to bring out any contrast between your nature and his."[3]

An interesting 1972 study showed men a group of pictures of women culled from all sorts of sources. There were naked centerfolds, women wearing bikinis, and others fully, sometimes elegantly dressed. The results were fascinating. Introverts liked their women to be thinner and more fully dressed; seemingly, they felt threatened by women who were too naked or too well endowed. They wanted "thin and thoughtful" females.

Manual workers wanted conventionally well-dressed women, and disliked those who wore 'trendy,' up-to-the-minute fashion. And when the men were asked which women they'd prefer as long-term mates, the male preferences moved toward *elegant, well-dressed* women, rather than the ones who were in sexy, provocative, nude, or semi-nude poses.[4]

Indeed, most of the sexy women I interviewed sensed this important preference, and nearly all told me that they avoid any necklines which are too low-cut, dresses that are high-slit or blatantly sexy.

A typical comment was, "I love to dress and feel feminine—ruffles (not many), lace, simple but elegant jewelry. I choose a dress or suit that allows me to be a 'total woman'! The unsexiest clothing bares the body inappropriately in comparison to those attending the occasion around you. For instance, men tend to love bare backs and low-cut tops/dresses, but not to the point that it leaves nothing for the imagination—especially in public. To 'gawk' alone with the one you love is one thing, but to have ten other men 'gawking' is another, especially if everything is totally visible and displayed for one and all."

Mandy Rice Davies, who was involved in the sexploits in the British Profumo scandal of the 60s, definitely could be described as a sexy woman. She has said, "If a woman wanted to project her 'good in bed' quality, I would always advise her to look nonsexy. Low-cut dresses seem out of date, and looking sexy is a very low-class turn-on. I don't think men are turned on in the flesh by overt sex. It is important to be a little more cool if you want to attract a glamorous man. The exploding iceberg bit works far better than looking sexy does."[5]

One man told me he prefers a woman "who is tastefully dressed, well-tailored. I don't really care for the bizarre or unusual. I'm not overly interested in plunging necklines—oh, if they are well done, showing just a little bosom, pretty conservative . . . but a woman shouldn't dress for attention. She should dress because she looks good, so that she projects a subtle, quiet effect."

Subtle is the key word. What types of clothing give that subtle promise of sexiness—without spoiling the effect by being too provocative? One of the most effective garments a woman can wear is a dress. Both men and women wear pants, but we never see men (except for female impersonators) in a dress. A dress, by its very style, is female.

Almost all of the men I surveyed said they found dresses either strongly sexy or moderately appealing, and nearly all the sexy women I talked to said they would choose a dress to wear for a first date with a man who was important to them. However, it was not just *any* dress, but one that made them feel sexy, elegant, special, and slightly understated.

"I like to wear clothes that do show what I look like," said Tracy, a top sales woman for her company. "Not blatant. One dress I have that I know is effective has red and white diagonal stripes, spaghetti straps, and it is almost a tent, except that it is on the bias and tends to cling. I have worn that dress to test whether or not a man appreciates what I have. It works great. I like clothes that move nicely."

Blatant turns off both men and women. Another woman told me that she would choose a dress that is "dressier than work, but not overly sexy. I don't want him to concentrate on the sexiness but on me. You don't have to broadcast sensuality. If you have to broadcast it, you might as well give it up."

"Sexy is classy," agreed a third. "I think it's more sexy to wear black that covers everything than it is to be gaudy—flashy. For instance on a dinner date I might wear a black dress with padded shoulders, something classy and sophisticated rather than showy and slinky."

As several women suggested, to have man-appeal a dress must hint at the body beneath and suggest movement. There is a poem I love (probably one reason is that it is about a woman named Julia). It was written by Robert Herrick, and touches upon the beauty of motion in clothing.

When as in silks my Julia goes,
Then, then, methinks, how sweetly flows
The liquefaction of her clothes!

Next, when I cast mine eyes and see
That brave vibration each way free,
—O how that glittering taketh me![6]

It is no accident that business suits generally have straight skirts—boxy, straight skirts are uninteresting and often lack sex appeal. Flared skirts, with their interesting play of swirly motion as the woman walks, are infinitely more sexual. Slinky pleats that move and shimmy are also sexy without being blatant.

As nearly every woman I talked to pointed out, a neckline does not have to be plunging to be sexual. What it does need is a suggestion of being slightly open, or a few buttons undone. Indeed, behaviorists for years have emphasized that a tight, high-buttoned neck indicates that the woman is "closed," whereas leaving a few buttons open indicates more openness.

When sexy women do want to get showy, they do it in understated ways. Said Terry, "I like to wear dresses that show off my waist, preferably with a full, maybe pleated skirt. I have one dress like that. It is in a pastel pattern, with a draped bow along one hip, and a "v" neckline that is fairly modest. I wore that to a dance one time and the effect was sensational. Even women were coming over to compliment me. I walked past three men who just dropped their conversation to stare at me—until I actually had to laugh. It was a total turn-on, that dress and the way I felt in it."

What other clothes appeal to men? Women who are selecting business suits to wear to work with the idea these will downplay their sexual attractiveness may be in for a surprise: Of the men I polled, more than 50 percent found business suits either strongly sexy or moderately appealing. This may be because the severity of the business uniform of the 1970s has relaxed, and now business garb has softened, both in color and in style.

Most of the men said they think bulky sweaters are moderately appealing, and about half also thought the very trendy, avant-garde fashion look to be appealing. (The remainder were cool on trendiness, finding the look either neutral or a turn-off.)

Men love to touch. Small boys love to stroke soft, cuddly materials like angora or rabbit fur, and big boys grow up to be just as tactile, loving the feel of a fabric as well as its look. Over and over, men have told me that they love soft-textured, touchable fabrics on women, and my survey bore this out. Nearly all of the men said they found soft-textured clothes either strongly sexy or moderately appealing.

The braless look still has strong appeal for men, although, to my surprise, about one-fourth said they found bralessness to be either neutral or a turn-off. Most of the men thought tight jeans were strongly sexy, again with a holdout of a few who found them a turn-off. Interestingly, the popularity of T-shirts is falling off, and, although one-fourth of the men thought them strongly sexy, another quarter thought T-shirts were either neutral or a turn-off.

As a curious by-way, I was once told by a man that he found panty-lines that show under a woman's clothes to be extremely sexy, so I included this question on my survey. I learned that although Madison Avenue may try to tell us that panty lines are a no-no, not all men find them to be so. In fact, 16 out of 73 men found panty-lines to be extremely sexy, and another nine found them moderately appealing!

Color choices are another fascinating phenomenon. Men definitely do have favorite shades. Priscilla Beaulieu Presley wrote about Elvis' clothes preferences: "He liked me in red, blue, turquoise, emerald green and black and white—the same colors he wore himself. He liked solids, declaring that prints were too distracting."[7]

When I asked men to name the colors they found most sexually appealing on women, the overwhelming favorite was red. Red is a provocative, sexy color, an all-or-nothing shade, the emotional color of fire, blood, excitement. It is chosen by women who are in the mood for excitement and who want to be found exciting—a challenge undoubtedly picked up on by men. I have heard women say that if they want to be asked to dance, they always wear red, and one women scribbled on her questionnaire that to be sexy she "wears red a lot."

The second favorite color of the men was black. We all know that black is sexy—but why? One color psychologist says that black is fascinating because it means surrender. "The white flag may be the international signal for military surrender, but when it comes to personal surrender it is *black* that creates that subconscious impression. Black implies sex appeal with a suggestion of sadness."[8]

And the men's third choice was white. White is sometimes

chosen by a sexy women who rejects red or black as being too blatantly obvious. White is the color of innocence, of demure virginity, and of lacy romanticism.

Earth tones may be fine for furniture, but women should avoid wearing them if they want to be sexy, according to the men I surveyed. When I asked men which colors they found to be least sexually appealing, the most disliked color was brown. This was followed by green, with pink, beige, and tan coming in behind. (Interestingly, the disliked brown tones are all shades that *men* choose a great deal, so perhaps they connotate maleness in the minds of these men.)

Men overwhelmingly loved black as their favorite shade in lingerie, black beating out all other shades, although 13 men said they did like red. The other colors so popular in lingerie shops, such as peach, nude, and white, received only token votes.

Larger Women

Although many of the men, in theory, found a woman more than 60 pounds overweight a turn-off, in real life the heavier woman can and does find partners. One woman of normal weight told me that she was thinking of writing a book called "Only the Fat Girls Get To Dance," because she'd seen so many heavy women having the time of their lives out on the dance floor.

The choices large women make are especially important in terms of how others view them. "Dressing fat," wearing lots of tents to cover the bulges, is a real killer to sex appeal.

Larger women do not have to give up a sexy look, say fashion experts who give hints for the woman who terms herself "big and beautiful." An all-of-a-color outfit is more slenderizing than is a hodgepodge of shades. And the look should go down to the toes, with encompassing shoes and hosiery as well.

Other tricks include plenty of vertical effects to fool the eyes, such as up-and-down stripes, lengthened cardigan jackets and v-necklines.

Emphasis at the neckline takes away from bulges elsewhere. This might includes capelets, scarves, large jewelry, and lovely collars that frame the face.

"One thing I do is choose *large* jewelry," says Kate, 33, who models larger-size fashions. "I mean, I walk into a store and I say, 'What's the biggest and the ugliest piece you've got?' That's the one I buy, and on me it looks proportional and very, very nice."

Skirt lengths vary but long, long skirts are not recommended for the heavier woman. As one fashion expert put it, "Lavishly laden ladies with parts that tend to pull downward do not require help in that direction." Pitfalls for the 14-plus wearer include tents ("If she's wearing a tent I figure it's only for one reason, to hide bulges," says one man) and any garment that is too tight.

Many of the men I surveyed said they disliked clothing that was too tight, a common mistake made by heavier women trying to get into clothes they've really outgrown. As one woman put it, "I'm one of these people who doesn't like to admit to myself that I've gained a little weight—so I keep on wearing the same clothes. Well, I had these jeans and even I had to admit they were too tight. I bought a larger size and do you know what? I had people come up to me and ask me if I'd lost weight. The new, larger jeans actually made me look slimmer than the tight ones."

Shoes

One aspect of sex appeal that many women overlook is—literally—right underfoot. I'm referring to the shoe. Rita Lydig was a wealthy socialite in the 1920s, a rich woman who collected hundreds of pairs of shoes, many made exclusively for her, and all of them outrightly sexy types. In 1970 the Metropolitan Museum of Art even prepared a special exhibit of them. She said, "In my view, sex begins with the foot. That's where a woman begins to dress up, or down. A shoe without sex appeal is like a tree without leaves—barren."[9]

One American shoe designer spoke bluntly about shoes. "But let's face it. The prime element we build into a woman's shoe is sex. If it lacks sex appeal, not only does it miss the mark of fashion, but it doesn't sell worth a damn. Shoes aren't merely sex symbols. They're sex motivators, because they help give a woman the look, the poise, the carriage, that conveys a sensual language."[10]

What qualities of a shoe make it sexy? The most important is the heel, according to William Rossi, author of *The Sex Life of the Foot and Shoe*. High heels give a woman a sexier, leggier look, making the arch and instep look more femininely curved. In fact, a three-inch heel will visually "shorten" a foot as much as two inches.

High heels do a lot more for a woman. They cause postural changes that accentuate voluptuousness in the pelvis, buttocks, curve of the back. They make the bosom look fuller, heavy legs appear thinner, and slim legs look curvier. High heels also feminize the gait by forcing a shortening of the stride, a more swaying, mincing step that suggests a degree of helpless bondage. There is a certain amount of sado-masochism, psychiatrists say, from the high heel that makes a woman less free, more dependent on masculine support.

Writes Susan Brownmiller: "The open-toed, high-heeled ankle strap with its sly imitation of a leg fetter, known in some quarters as the fuck-me shoe, is another variation on love-slave eroticism . . . "[11]

High heels also add to the height of the wearer, giving her a psychological and emotional uplight, equally important in sex appeal. Have you ever seen a beauty queen in flat heels, or a professional stripper? High heels make the difference as to whether a burlesque queen is simply a naked woman on stage or a voluptuous and sexy one.

Most of the men I surveyed said they thought "very high heels" were very sexy or moderately appealing, although about 10 considered the "very" to be excessive.

A skin-tight fit is another very-sexy attribute of certain shoes, Rossi says, because the snug fit accents foot shape and the sinuous movement of the foot inside. Materials that are sensuous include some of the softer leathers such as kidskin and calfskin.

A pointed or tapered toe is far sexier than a round or stubby toe, which always desexualizes a shoe. Bright colors shout out sexuality. And seminakedness in a shoe—like strippy sandals, low-cut shell pumps, cutouts over the vamp, or deepcut throat-lines that expose toe lines—can be a real turn-on.

The throatline of a shoe, incidentally, is the top part, just below the instep, and it is called that because of the similarity between this and the bosom's larger cleavage. "There are many different types of throatlines on women's shoes, but, significantly, *never* on men's shoes," says Rossi. "On the shoe, as on the dress, the shape of the throatline can be low-cut or high-cut, V-shaped, round, or square. A sexy dress exposes bosom cleavage. A sexy shoe exposes toe cleavage."[12]

It is no coincidence that talk of shoes often brings out sensuous language like *cleavage* and *naked*. There is all sorts of eroticism in shoes. One man told me about his girlfriend who bought a new pair of shoes that were decorated with little slits along the edge of the throatline. Both of them stared down at the shoes for a while, he related; her skin was showing through the slits. "Finally she looked down at that shoe and smiled, and said, 'That looks like lots of little pussies,' and, yeah, she was right. It did, and do you know what? It was really sexy. Those shoes were really a turn-on."

If high heels are sexy, flat heels definitely are not. Most of the men I surveyed found flat heels to be either neutral or a turn-off. The most sexless shoes in the trade are known by such names as "sensible," or "comfort," or even "old ladies' running shoes." What is a sexless shoe? It has a low or flat heel, a mannish oxford or tie style, a rounded or bulbous toe. Its color is black or some other dull, drab color.

However, many women choose something in between, something comfortable and not extreme, going by a name that Rossi terms "neuter." "Neuter" shoes are just that—neither sexy nor sexless. They are conservative fashion, known in the trade as "mama" and "dumb" shoes.

"Neuter shoes reflect a quiescent or semiactive libido," insists Rossi. "When a woman, especially a married one with a growing family, passes age forty or so, she often gets into the habit of wearing neuter-type shoes. Her concern is to dress 'nicely' as she thinks a middle-aged wife and mother should. She's no longer sending sex signals to other men."[13]

Hair

Hairstyles are another very strong way that women send out sexual signals to men. Linda Stasi, in her book, *Looking Good*

Is the Best Revenge, catalogs hair styles in terms of sex appeal. Short, cropped hair conveys a no-nonsense image that implies the wearer is more concerned with what she is doing than how she looks doing it. Hair pulled back into a bun or tight pony tail shows cool-headed conservatism. It contributes to a look that men call "tight"—the exact opposite of sexiness.

If you wear bangs that cover most of your forehead, you may be pulling back from the world, giving the impression that you're shy, or just don't have the confidence to face people straight on. (And remember, showing *confidence* is vital for sex appeal.)

Wearing hair *too neatly* is another killer of sex appeal, sending out strong "stay away" messages. Tight, immaculate grooming without a hair out of place indicates a tightly controlled, powerfully self-disciplined individual. At the next cocktail party you attend, look around: Who is the woman who is receiving the most attention from men? It won't be the woman whose hair looks as if it's enclosed in Lucite. "That scares people away," says Stasi, "Because it makes you look unfriendly, untouchable, and untenable."[14]

Listen to what one sexy woman says about her hair: "I blow-dry my hair—it's shoulder length—and I like it really messy. I think it's a lot more sexy to have it messy, wild, natural-looking, some of it more on one side. When the wind comes, the hair shifts twice, it's flowing, natural, and you don't get bothered if someone rolls down the car window."

Poet Robert Herrick had something to say about untidiness, too. He wrote in the 1600s, but his eye for a sexy woman was unerring, and his ideas about the "delight in disorder" are still valid today.

> *A sweet disorder in the dress*
> *Kindles in clothes a wantonness:*
> *A Lawn about the shoulders thown*
> *Into a fine distraction:*
> *An erring lace, which here and there*
> *Enthralls the crimson stomacher:*
> *A cuff neglectful, and thereby*
> *Ribbons to flow confusedly:*
> *A winning wave (deserving note)*
> *In the tempestuous petticoat:*

A careless shoe-string, in whose tie
I see a wild civility:
Do more bewitch me, than when art
Is too precise in every part.[15]

Even in the sport of female body building, women contestants are forced to consider the signals their hair sends to the male judges. Says Lydia Cheng, a top bodybuilder, "Rightly or wrongly, the sport emphasizes sex appeal and a lot of women use that sex-kitten image to get points, since most of the judges are men." One bodybuilder, Rachel McLish, known for her sexy, wild-woman locks, says she feels hair is as important as the body. "It's a wild-woman look that the male judges fantasize about and the female judges live vicariously through."[16]

What types of hair do men like best? A recent survey of 1,000 men conducted by Procter & Gamble's Ivory Shampoo and Conditioner division focused on male hair loves and hates— most of which were also borne out by my survey. Eighty-eight percent of the Procter & Gamble men liked medium to long hair. "It makes a woman seem romantic," was a typical comment. Only 10 percent of the Procter & Gamble men liked short hair, on the other hand, with men from New York City disliking short tresses most vehemently. "Businesslike and unfeminine" was their decree.[17]

What about shades? Blondes won top billing in my survey as "most appealing," and 35 percent of the Procter & Gamble men put blonde hair first. Dr. Joyce Brothers has made it clear that she intends to stay a blonde forever, saying she believes that blondes attract more men because men think of blondes as fun dates. The woman who is treated warmly and flirtaciously reacts warmly and flirtaciously—and, as Dr. Brothers adds, "life gets lighter and brighter along with her hair."

But 29 percent of the Procter & Gamble men liked brown hair, 13 percent liked red hair, and 10 percent black hair. And gray? Only 1 percent of the P. & G. men preferred gray hair on women, but of the men I surveyed, the men were much more tolerant. Of the 73 men, 38 said gray hair "wasn't important," and 9 found it "fairly appealing."

Curls? More than half of the P. & G. men liked soft waves, considering them more feminine, but 17 percent did go for curls, and 21 percent of the men preferred straight hair.

Long hair on women has long been considered provocative or erotic, especially by strait-laced societies such as that of the Puritans, who solved the problem of too much sexiness by making women cover their hair with a hat or other pious headgear, or roll it into a tight knot.

But whatever the color or hairstyle, men want a woman's hair to be *soft*. Sexy women sense this. One woman told me, "I always get a lot of compliments on my hair. Guys like it if the hair is softer. I have thick, curly, fairly soft hair. Guys touch it sometimes—to me that is sexy. I had one man say while I was dancing with him what soft hair I had, and he wanted to know what I washed it with, it smelled so clean and nice and fresh. My hair isn't full of hair spray, I can't stand that. All I do is wash it and pick it—that's it. And I use a soft, soft creme rinse—men really like that."

Hair spray or mousse is a turn-off to most men. It unconsciously signals that the wearer is stiff, tense, and doesn't want to be touched. Said one man, "It's sexy to me to be able to take my hand and stroke the back of a woman's neck, there's such a soft, silky feel, I get all excited over that. But I hate hair spray. Some women think they look nice, and maybe it's okay for a picture, say, but I've seen women who look like they have a schaum torte on their head. That's a cake with egg white on it and strawberries underneath. It looks all fluffed up and it's hard and crusty. Hair spray is a crusty top. When you touch it the hair is not alive. I like hair to be soft and pliable, so it moves."

By the way: about glasses. Women who worry that men won't make passes, will be pleasantly surprised to learn that eyeglasses weren't necessarily a turn-off to three-quarters of the men I polled. They said that if a woman wore glasses it "wasn't important" to their view of her sex appeal—and 13 of the men actually said that they found glasses appealing!

Make-up

One of the most effective ways women have of sending out sexual signals is through the use of make-up—as the cosmetics industry has been telling us for decades. But cosmetics are more than just prettification. They capitalize on unconscious sex awareness. For instance, take eyeliner. One effect of eyeliner is to accentuate the darkness of our pupils, to make them seem larger and more dilated. (Pupil dilation is one of the physiological signs of sexual arousal.)

But most people notice dilated pupils only on an unconscious level. Indeed, psychologists have discovered that men, over and over, will chose a picture of a woman whose pupils have been retouched to look larger. Fashion photographers often retouch their model's pictures, to achieve this same, sexy effect!

Blush lends a sexual flush to the cheeks, and the sheen that moisturizer and foundation give to the skin mimics that healthy, perspiring glow a woman's skin gets during and after the act of making love. Shiny red lips are a sexual attractant, imitating, as they do, the healthy red-pink of a woman's genital area. Red lips appear full, warm, pouty, alluring, while pale lips seem drawn and anxious, far less attractive.

Make-up has another interesting effect, too—it makes people more easily remember what you say. Researchers at Scripps College in Claremont, California, made three video tapes using a 20-year-old college student. All the tapes, "starring" the same woman were identical except for one thing—the star's make-up. In one tape, she wore little, and looked very plain. In another tape, she was made up to look average. And in the third, make-up was applied to make the student look as gorgeous as possible. Then the video tapes were shown to three groups of 50 men and women. Result: The more attractively made up the woman was, the more accurately both men and women remembered what she said![18]

One man I interviewed for the book, a 48-year-old salesman, seemed fascinated by my survey form with its questions on make-up preferences. A few days later he called to tell me, "I kept thinking about your questions on make-up, and today I happened to go to the bank, and I was looking around at all the tellers. I kept trying to pinpoint which tellers I was looking at the most. And finally I figured it out—it was the ones who had the most make-up on. They were the ones I was looking at."

Sexy women may rate far above average in their use of make-up. A recent *Ladies Home Journal* survey of 102,000 readers revealed that only 44.7 percent spend at least fifteen minutes or more a day putting make-up on.[19] Fifteen minutes is not very long, especially if make-up is applied several times in the day. However, of the sexy women I surveyed, nearly *all* said they wear make-up nearly always, and the remainder said they wore it most of the time.

But there is a strange contradiction here. Sexy women do wear make-up. And yet, for men *wearing too much make-up* is almost a universal turn-off, and one man felt so strongly about this that he equated the wearing of too much make-up in the same general category as drug-taking and alcoholism! There is a telling word men often use to describe women who are wearing what the man thinks is too much make-up-- and that word is *hard.*

Once I attended an annual party with a male friend, and afterward my escort told me that one of the women looked "hard." I was startled, for the previous year a different escort had said exactly the same thing about the same woman. I'd known Cathy, in trim middle age, for years and she is a sweet, warm, and loving woman. What on earth could have caused these men to think her hard? But after a bit of thinking I realized what it was. Cathy, in her late 50s, had overdone the make-up, even to the extent of wearing fake eyelashes.

But this dichotomy about "hardness" and make-up is easily solved: No matter how much make-up a woman really is wearing, men want her to *look* as if she's wearing only a light amount. This may date back, as Susan Brownmiller speculates, to the old Hollywood vamps and sirens, and the stereotype no-good woman of the silent film, who wore heavy eye make-up and lip paint to indicate destructive sexuality. (And as "wicked" women on the evening soaps still do to this day.)

As one male college student related, "Wearing too much make-up is a real turn-off to me. One girl didn't wear it when I met her, and then when I went out with her she trundled on the make-up." What did "trundling" mean, I asked? "When it kind of flakes off."

Another man's definition of heavy make-up was, "gaudy, heavy eyeshadow, heavy rouge beyond bright, standoutish, and really, really red lipstick."

Most men like light make-up. Of the men I surveyed, nearly all said they found it either "extremely appealing," or "fairly appealing." In fact, half found *no* makeup "fairly appealing," and one man told me that he had gone with his grilfriend for three months before he realized that she wore no makeup!

But what about the gorgeous, heavily made-up magazine face, the one we see on the cover of *Cosmo* and in the ads for companies like Coty and Revlon? Men don't necessary go for the face that is engineered with cosmetics. In fact, of the men I polled, *more than half* said they thought lots of make-up, like a magazine model, was *a turn-off.*

Perfumes can also indicate sexuality. More than half of the sexy women I talked to wear perfume "nearly always," and most of the rest "usually." The majority of men find perfume or cologne "fairly appealing," with one-fourth saying they find it "extremely appealing." Several qualified their vote by mentioning that it all depended on "how much," and "on whom."

One masseur said that he is fully aware of the hedonistic effect of scents on sexuality and carefully avoids using perfumes in his work. "Scented aids arouse my patients, men and women. I just can't handle that. I use a very light mineral oil, warmed up, and I don't use scents anywhere in my studio!"

Perfume is most effective when placed on the pulse points of the body, says Annette Green, executive director of the Fragrance Foundation. These places—at the bend of the elbow, wrists, behind the knees, the bosom, and base of the throat—are warmer because the blood flows closest to the skin. Another sexy place to spray perfume is on clean hair. Green herself says she likes to apply it to the palms of her hands so the fragrance can release itself as she moves.

However, like any good thing, perfume can be overdone so as to reach the turn-off point. As Sydney J. Harris once quipped, "A woman who uses too much perfume is only calling attention to her need for it."

Subtle Signals

Last year I was a guest on a radio call-in show in Denver, Colorado. At 2 AM, a woman called in with a plaintive and heartfelt question. She had been reading a magazine article about the Yale-Harvard report, we discussed in an earlier chapter, that was filled with scary statistics about how a never-married woman over the age of 30 has only a slight chance of marrying. She herself was 30 years old, a working woman, she told me, of normal weight for her height, and she said, "I don't look bad. Really I don't. And I want to get married sometime."

Yet she was having problems. "All the men are coming on to me as buddies," she explained to me over the air. "They don't want to take me out on a date, they just want to be friends. I don't want to spend the rest of my life like this. . . . That article scares me. I don't want to believe it. Yet all the men want to be to me is buddies. What's wrong?"

On the radio, you have only a few seconds to respond with some short, pithy piece of wisdom. Even after I gave the woman her answer (maybe she was unconsciously dressing like someone's aunt, rather than a lover, and maybe she should let her hair grow longer), I still pondered. Surely there must be millions of women in this predicament. Over 30, puzzled, a little scared, yearning, yet not knowing how to reach out and grasp the sex appeal that could be theirs.

As I worked on this book, this woman kept coming to my mind, and finally I decided to ask the men and women I interviewed about her problem. What should a woman do when she is of normal weight for her height, of average appearance, but the men only come on to her as buddies?

Their answers were surprisingly helpful.

The most common response from both sexes was this one: *She needs to change her signals. Somehow she's signalling men that this is all she wants—buddies, not lovers.*

"The messages she's sending out say she's available on those terms, accessible on those terms, only as a buddy," responded one man. "She presents herself in nonsexual terms. She could dress differently, be more suggestive, could figure out how to present herself as more available. It depends a lot on the kinds of things she does. Most women I dance with dance far back, kind of away from me. She could get real cuddly. If she's dancing far back, she's not encouraging a relationship."

The woman should be careful how she *starts* a relationship with a man, cautioned another man. If a relationship starts on a friendly basis, then that's how it's likely to continue. "The other person will come back as a friend most of the time and not cross that line."

Bill, 26, agreed. "She's doing something to make herself appear sisterlike to these men. She's putting up boundaries, like she probably sits further away in the car, she doesn't look at them when they're talking, she does negative things. She has to do something to her thinking that will project in her actions. When she admits what she wants and that she's good enough to deserve it, and when she believes it, all those things will change."

She Should Act More Feminine.   Most of the men and women I talked to pointed out that acting like "one of the boys" is a fatal error.

"Girls who go out drinking with the guys all the time or who want to play softball and not do their nails. . . . they do get branded as one of the guys. Put a little make-up on, and don't talk like the guys either," advised Bob, one single man. He, along with others, suggested that she not participate in the rough, rowdy male cameraderie. "Point out things to them, like if they are using bad language in front of her. Tell them it rubs her the wrong way."

One of the sexy women I talked to agreed that using feminine-type language is very important. "She shouldn't talk like a man, she should talk like a woman if she wants something different. At times she will have to leave the conversation. You don't stay if it's real male conversation, if they're talking about women and getting real rowdy, that's my opinion."

Most of the sexy women agreed that our 30-year-old woman should make more feminine choices in dress and hair style. "This woman at work who has the same problem always wears her hair real short," one pointed out. "She could do a lot to make herself look softer and different. My sister, too, could look much softer. The one thing about her that would make a real difference is that she has these very strong, big eyebrows, and that makes her hard-looking."

"I have one outfit," says a blonde sales manager of 46, "And when I wear it, there is no *way* a man could think of me as a buddy. It has a black skirt with a black lace bottom, and

I wear a black leotard and strap shoes—I get many compliments on that outfit. I would wear that with someone I thought of as a good buddy, show them a side of me they're not aware of. Get the conversation into a realm that's a little bit suggestive. I've done that, too."

She Should Portray Herself as a Potential Sex Partner.
Pointed out one handsome 29-year-old engineer, the problem with our 30-year-old is that she is not making the moves. "Men are basically chicken, they are too scared of rejection. If she wants more she should indicate more, especially in the workplace. It's scary at times for a man, in the workplace, to make it more than buddies."

She should go places where the emphasis is on dating, to show that that's what she's interested in. "If I were that woman," remarked Jeanne, "I would take a good look at the places where I went. I'd try organizations where you could be assured the men were out looking for dates and were not married. At a typical nightclub too many of the men are either married or alcoholics. I've been to a lot of them but I've rarely come across a good prospect even for dating. People criticise Parents Without Partners and groups like that, but at least everyone is divorced and has had relationships, so they're capable of having them, they're more likely to be at least interested in dating."

She May Be Scaring Men Off by Being Too Needy—Wanting to Get Married Too Much.
She's probably trying too hard, pointed out one college professor. "She's obviously giving off the wrong cues, and not communicating a sexual interest. Maybe she scares hell out of the men. One of my colleagues is interested in marriage, and the men pick up on this. This can be very constraining, and will scare a man off faster than anything."

A woman agreed. "She probably comes off as wanting to get married and this scares men off. I knew a woman like that. She was really pretty, she had a Connecticut–New England look, blonde and so forth, but maybe she was too friendly and nice—she was always available, too available. A woman should act more in demand."

Others agreed she should act more mysterious, harder to

get. "Maybe," said one woman, "She should be more independent. How? You don't hang around a man, you walk away when he wants to see more of you."

She Should Invite her Male "Buddies" Out on a Real Date.
"If these men are buddies," remarked Ken, 33, "All she has to do is issue an invitation, come up with tickets to something, ask them out. She's already got the perfect setup—namely that these men are friends."

Start doing things together that are fun, advised another man. "Not necessarily expensive, but things like going to the zoo, where you can buy peanuts and feed the bears, walk and talk and maybe touch a little. Touching is so important, to grab the arm and tease, a hug around the shoulders, a little body language that says 'relax around me.'"

"She'll have to say, call me up next week and let's go for dinner and dancing," said a woman. "Put herself on a different level, not go out for beer, but let's get dressed up."

She Should Develop Flirting and Talking Skills.   Perhaps our dateless 30-year-old is rusty in her flirting skills or in the way she talks to men. "Something is missing," one man pronounced. "It could be something screwball, like having bad teeth, or a cigarette dangling out of her mouth. But if the guys want to be buddies, then she is distancing them, not being soft and friendly. It could be what she talks about. Maybe her conversation is masculine-oriented, she talks only sports and business, that would do it. Or if she was unwilling to reveal any of her feelings."

One man gave graphic hints on how the woman could psych herself into working on her attitude. "While in the company of a man she'd like to attract, I'd advise her to actively think, 'I want you to fuck me. I want to feel your cock inside of me. I want to drive you wild in bed.' The obscenity is not gratuitous—I sincerely feel that the harshness of such thoughts may well carry over in all sorts of telling ways."

"I hate to sound sexist," added a woman, "but it might help if a woman acts like she depends on a man. If she can do everything for herself, he might think she doesn't need a lover. She should act as if she appreciates some of the male-type of things he can do for her."

***She Should Count herself Lucky that She Does Have all Those
Male Friends.***   Several of my interviewees mentioned this.
"Most women would find it very attractive that they would be
considered as a buddy, they are three steps ahead rather than
behind," pointed out a 42-year-old financial planner.

Many women agreed. "If I had a choice between men carrying on for sex, or as buddies, I'd choose buddies every time,"
said one attactive 29-year-old woman whose cloud of dark curls
is very fetching. "She has some signals, she's letting them know
that that's what she wants."

But as one man reassured, the woman *was* looking, and
that was most important. "She should keep right on looking
until what she is looking for is what the other one is looking
for, a harmony."

Axioms of Sex Appeal

1. Every time we put clothing on our body, or do something to our
   bodies, we are sending out a signal to others: This is who I am,
   and I've chosen this article to show you. Each time you get
   dressed in the morning you are sending out messages to men
   as to how confident you are, how sexy you feel.

2. When thinking about a long-term relationship, men prefer women
   who dress well and elegantly, studies have found. Most sexy
   women sense this and avoid choosing clothing that is too blatantly sexy. The secret is being *subtle*.

3. The most effective clothing a woman can wear is a dress. In the
   first place, a dress is not worn by men. All of the sexy women
   said they would choose a dress to wear on a first date with someone who was important to them. And nearly all the men said
   they found a dress either strongly sexy or moderately appealing.

4. Business suits are not always brush-offs to sexual attractiveness,
   as some women may think, especially with today's more relaxed
   styles. More than half of the men I polled found suits either
   strongly sexy or moderately appealing.

5. Men love soft-textured fabrics and find them sensuously appealing.

6. Tight jeans and the braless look still have their appeal for men,
   although the popularity of T-shirts is falling off.

7. Surprisingly, although Madison Avenue tells us that showing "panty lines" under clothing is a no-no, some men do find panty lines to be sexy.

8. Red is the color that men find most sexually appealing on women, followed by black and then—a lagging third choice—white. Women should avoid wearing earth tones if they want to be sexy. The men most disliked the color brown, followed by green, with pink, beige and tan also in disfavor. Perhaps the reason men don't like the browns and beiges is that these are shades usually worn by men.

9. Although most of the men I surveyed said they found a woman more than 60 pounds overweight a turn-off, in real life many larger women do find partners. "Dressing fat" is a real killer to sex appeal, and the larger woman must dress to complement her good points, to minimize her weight.

10. Shoes are an aspect of sex appeal that many women overlook. Actually, shoes can send out strong sexual messages. The sexiest shoes are those with heels, because high heels visually "shorten" the foot and cause postural changes that emphasize sexual characteristics. Skin-tight shoes are sexy, as are those with a pointed or tapered toe, or a low-cut throatline that emphasizes "toe cleavage." Bright colors emphasize sex appeal.

11. The sexiest hair style is one that looks flyaway, loose and soft. Wearing the hair too neatly kills sexiness, giving out strong "stay away" messages. Men like long, wavy hair and blonde hair, and many say gray hair "isn't important."

12. Make-up makes a woman more noticeable, and people are more apt to remember what she says. However, men think that wearing "too much make-up" is a turn-off, and prefer a woman to look as if she is wearing a light amount. Half of the men I talked to said they found it appealing when a woman wore no make-up.

13. If a man isn't making sexual advances, but is rather coming on to a woman as a buddy, she should examine the signals she is sending out and make changes. Somehow she is signalling men that she doesn't want a lover. She should act more feminine and portray herself as potential partner, going places where the emphasis is on dating. She should try inviting her male "buddies" out on a date, act less needy, and develop flirting and talking skills.

10

Turn-ons and Turn-offs

It is about as stupid to let your clothes betray that you know you are ugly as to have them proclaim that you know you are beautiful.

—Edith Wharton

If a mythical genie were to appear in front of you right now and offer to grant you only one wish in regard to your sex appeal, what would that wish be? Would you wish for a sexier body, for blonder hair, to be shorter, taller, cuter, larger breasted?

If you wish for those items, you may be making a mistake because, according to the men I talked to, the most common turn-on in sex appeal is *confidence*. Over and over these men told me that even if the woman lacks a pefect body, her sexual confidence will carry her through.

"I can go into a room and tell within a couple of minutes who's sexy and who isn't," announced one man as I interviewed him in the clubhouse of a local golf course. A women's league happened to be filling up the tables in the long room, clusters of women laughing together and comparing scores.

"All right," I challenged. "Who's sexy in this room?"

He glanced around the room for about 25 seconds. "Okay. There's only one woman in this room I consider sexy." He pointed to a woman about 41 years old, a slim brunette, who was talking animatedly with her friends. "See her? The way she sits, the way she holds her head? She's interested in the conversation, she's involved, she's not withdrawn into herself, too much focused on her own interests. She looks confident about herself."

Confidence was mentioned again and again. "Women have to be straight with themselves," one 26-year-old attorney insisted. "Confidence is so attractive. I have discovered that I like a woman who doesn't really need you. She wants you in her life but she has other interests, other things that are important, too. I hate it when you've been going with a woman for two months or so, and suddenly you're the center of her life, around which everything else revolves."

Good grooming was another strong turn-on (just as the women who gave definitions of sex appeal in chapter one suspected.) Repeatedly men expressed aversion to such gross no-no's as "hairy pits," "unshaven legs," "no stockings," "dirty hair," and "body odor."

A few men mentioned body types they preferred, or focused on items such as "sexy clothing" or "dressing provocatively." But most of the men, when asked what things a woman could do to attract their sexual interest, named *personality qualities.*

Here are some qualities the men listed as turn-ons:

- Having confidence
- Being happy
- Smiling
- Being neat and well-turned-out
- Looking in good physical condition
- Being adventuresome
- Being a toucher and a hugger
- Being a good listener
- Wearing sexy undergarments
- Wearing bright colors

Another big attractant is when women show strong interest in a man. Many men found a woman's interest in them irresistable, saying that they find themselves drawn to a woman who likes them, even if her body is not perfect.

"I'd advise a woman to listen to me, to focus her undivided attention upon me, to go out of her way to make me feel special, unique, interesting," says one good-looking male writer in his 30s. "At heart, I believe that most men never lose the rather immature desire to be the center of attention. Come to think of it, most women enjoy occupying center stage as well."

Intelligence is another strong come-on for many men who stress, even in their definition of sex appeal, that it has to include some brains. This preference goes all the way from college students to men in their 50s and 60s. One October I had gone to visit my 20-year-old son, at Miami University in Oxford, Ohio. We were having lunch in a campus coffee shop while, outside the plate glass window, a veritable parade of blonde, corn-fed coeds strutted past in Miami University sweatshirts.

Something made me ask, "What kind of women do you like, Michael?" I was expecting an answer along the lines of, "Oh, blondes, Mom."

Instead the reply I got was, "Intelligent women, Mom. Like you." Later in his apartment I discussed this further with Michael and his two roommates, and all three emphatically agreed. Intelligence was their standard in women, and it was a standard they often found difficult to meet, even in a university setting.

Older men, the ones who responded to my survey, were just as firm. "I want a woman who has developed a broad range of interests, someone you can talk to who can talk back," emphasized a 38-year-old engineer. "She reads the newspapers, that's important, otherwise I can't relate. The other stuff, sexiness, is nice for lighting the fire, but to fuel the fire you have to have intelligence, lots of interest, someone you can talk to."

"I'm turned off by stupid women," said a teacher emphatically. "I know that many men find naive, ingenuous women appealing, but they turn my stomach. If a woman wants to excite me, she should allow her intellect to show through clearly. Intelligence enhances a woman's sex appeal by announcing that here's a bright, sophisticated, capable woman who knows what she wants and how to get it. She expects to take as much as she receives."

Other qualities named included playfulness, spontanaeity, being a good listener, being warm, being a toucher and a hugger, and not being afraid to talk about her feelings.

"I want a woman to be adventuresome," announced one single man. "Like, let's say she lives in another city and I call her up and say, 'I'm going to be in town and I need a place to stay.' She'll say, yes, she knows some good places to go. . . . I like it that she knows a little about things already, she's not looking to you to show her around. Or I might say I want to go and hear some polyphonic madrigals. She wouldn't say, 'Forget it, that sounds weird,' She'd want to try it out."

Another man agreed. He has been single for about six years now, searching for a relationship that will meet his needs. One night, over drinks, he began telling me how hard it was to find a woman who wanted to *do* things. "You'd be surprised how hard it is to find a woman who has just a little spirit of adventure in her," he said. "I'm interested in finding someone who might want to go up in a hot-air balloon with me, or go roller skating, or maybe even go to a tractor pull, a drag-boat race, something a little bit different. Most women over 35 just aren't into those things, they want the standard dinner out by candlelight. I've really found it very disappointing."

Hints from Sexy Women

The women I talked to were pragmatic in their ideas on how to be sexy, focusing on doing sexy little things for yourself, and on keeping your appearance and clothing male-noticeable. Here are some samples:

- "Every time you leave the house, always dress, even if you're just going shopping. I always have on lipstick and a little blush. Don't go anyplace with curlers, don't look too tacky. When you do see a good-looking man, if you're too tacky he won't look at you."

- "Do sports. It gives you freer movements, better muscle tone, a sexier body. Play sports to play well and create a good body more than to win. Sore winners, worse than sore losers, are a pain in the butt to everyone. I loved reading somewhere that most sports, like tennis, are an agreement to cooperate rather than a chance to destroy. And I like to think of sexual relationships in the same way."

- "Buy clothes that are you. A lot of women buy clothes that aren't really meant for them, and it shows. Wear clothes that make you feel good, not necessarily to attract men, but to make you feel good. You'll come across as confident, feminine, sexy."

- "Carry yourself with confidence. Walk like you are special to you, confident to yourself."

- "Do little things for yourself, like wear sexy underwear just to know you've got it on, so you feel that you are sexy underneath."

❧ "If you have time before a date, rather than taking a shower, take a bath before you go out. When I take a bubble bath and shave my legs, it makes me feel at my best. It's very relaxing and makes you feel more feminine."

❧ "Keep your hair clean and neat, and if you color it, keep it up—there's nothing worse than black roots. I think real long, straggly hair on older women looks cheap."

❧ "Smoking is unsexy."

❧ "Wear clothes that accent your shape a little. Box types show that you have looks you're trying to hide. Even though you might be wearing a loose type blouse, you should wear a little belt with it to show off your waistline. The boxy look doesn't hide anything, all it does is tell that you're trying to hide bulges."

❧ "Don't wear too much make-up—the men don't like it when they kiss someone who's wearing an inch of lipstick. If you have nice eyes, wear make-up in a tasteful way. And blend blush in. I hate to see this red line across a woman's face, it makes her look like a clown. Blend it so it doesn't show, feather it across the cheeks into the hairline, it looks much more becoming and gives you a glow."

❧ "Men like women with painted fingernails. More men I've been out with have said, 'Why don't you do your fingernails?' At least four or five men have told me that."

❧ "Try to wear some kind of make-up when you go out, especially at night when darkness fades everything. You do need to do *something* if you want to attract any kind of attention at all. If I didn't wear any make-up I could look very rugged. I'm a redhead and I have to tone down my complexion. If I didn't wear any mascara I would have gold eyelashes."

❧ "I don't think a woman should have beer on the first date, she should choose a more feminine drink. Something so that he'll think, she's not like him."

❧ "Men like great bodies, and a little bit longer hair, it's true. They like women who dance with them, who make it easy for them to dance. Who let them talk. Who are warm and easy and smile a lot. If a woman is warm and happy and confident, men feel at ease."

Turn-offs

Turn-offs to sex appeal are as varied as men are, and some of them are idiosyncratic. Also, what turns off one man might be a turn-on to another. I was struck by the questionnaire I distributed, when, no matter what body type I named, some men found it appealing, while others said it was a turn-off.

Still, over and over, my interviews turned up some common male dislikes, repeated often enough to be worth listening to. Some of my readers may look over these lists and feel amused— who, they ask, could actually be committing these slovenly sins, which read like a list of all the things our mothers told us *never* to do. But yes, Virginia, apparently thousands of women are doing them, and, by so doing, robbing themselves of sex appeal.

To be sexy is to send out messages to other people. Most turn-offs are also messages—negative ones. Men are incredibly good at picking up on these messages, and not only that, at looking beyond the small turn-off to see how it fits into a larger category that tells something important about the woman.

Looking over the list, most sins against sexinessness fall into eight basic categories. (And, by the way, these turn-offs are phrased in male language, just the way they were given to me.)

I Don't Care.   There are some things a woman does that indicate—loudly and clearly—that she doesn't consider herself sexy, doesn't want to be sexy, and be damned to anyone who might even put her in that category. By committing these sins, she is telling the world that her body isn't important to her, nor is it important that others look on her with admiration. Following is a list of qualities applicable to these women:

- Slovenliness
- Dirty appearance
- Bad breath
- Make-up on the collar

- Sloppy hair
- Body odor
- Unshaven legs
- Hairy pits
- No stockings
- Frumpy appearance (messy)

An occasional grooming lapse may be forgiven—but when a man sees a woman perhaps only once, at a market or a party, he has no way of knowing if this is a lapse or a permanent condition.

Kay is an example of a woman who doesn't even try to enter the competition. I saw Kay at the supermarket pushing a basket, clad in a pair of rumpled, dirty shorts and an old, much-washed T-shirt. Kay's hair had been cut any old which-way, and hadn't seen the benefit of permanent wave, curlers or curling iron—it just hung. She wore old, scuffed sandals, and her feet were dirty, her toenails long and ragged-looking. Need I say more? No man on the lookout for a sexy woman would give Kay a second glance—which may be exactly what she unconsciously wants.

Poor Self-Esteem.   This is one turn-off category that really bothers men and is a quick and instant deterrant to sex appeal. Men quickly spot a woman who doesn't feel good about herself, and they translate that rather lumpy, slumpy, hangdog look as "not sexy." Since most men consider high self-esteem to be part and parcel of sexiness to start with, any indication of the opposite being true is repugnant to them.

Here are some turn-offs men named in this category:

- Overweight
- Bad posture
- Eyes sunken, lack of sparkle
- Lack of confidence
- Basic, white, cotton underwear
- Low self-esteem
- Passivity

- Women who don't make any effort to be attractive
- Lack of muscle tone-- flab
- Dumpy, 'I don't care about my looks' look

Lois has poor self-esteem and it shows. Everything about Lois looks de-energized and slow. The color of her skin is pasty, as if she seldom exercises, and she walks at a rather slow, shoulders-bent pace, looking down at the ground. Lois isn't overweight—a doctor would probably say that she shows up "normal" on the weight charts. But she has poor muscle tone and, especially with her poor posture, her stomach protrudes in a little round belly. Her breasts, too, sag and appear smaller than they really are. Lois also chooses drab, fade-into-the-woodwork clothes in shades of beige and tan, generally wearing them loose.

Men look past Lois because she projects a sort of hangdog look that turns them off. What they are interested in is energy, vivacity, confidence, bounce—qualities that Lois' poor self-esteem won't let her have.

Trying Too Hard.   Ironically, trying too hard and too desperately to be sexy has just the opposite effect. Men don't want a woman to seem desperate or needy, especially when it comes to sex appeal, because if a woman has to try too hard, that means she *isn't* sexy. Men are extremely intuitive at picking up messages of this sort, too. Trying too hard covers a variety of sins, everything from "putting on an act," to "acting too cute." Here are some turn-offs named by men:

- Putting on an act
- Acting coy
- Aggressiveness
- Being too thin
- Being materialistic
- Being too provocative
- Wearing clothes too tight
- Coming on too strong
- Being overdressed

- Being overly cute
- Having big mouths
- Using inappropriate seductive behavior
- Talking too much

Overt aggressiveness is especially disliked by men. In sexual attraction, one of the unspoken requirements is for the female to let the male know that it is safe to approach her. When women are *too* aggressive, , this interferes with the whole process. One of the most blatant examples of aggressiveness I ever saw was several years ago, when a group of unattached singles went out together after a dance for a late-night breakfast. One woman, Angie, was sitting between two men, each of whom had ordered fried eggs.

Picking up her fork, Angie deliberately leaned over and punctured the two yolks belonging to the man on her right. As he stared at her, startled at this invasion of his space (and his food), the man to Angie's left hunched over his plate, protecting his eggs with his hands. Not only did this women aggressively invade these men's space, symbolically she also punctured their masculine "balls"!

Putting on an act is also trying too hard, and men sense this. Any woman who plays too coy, or too cute, or any other thing that she's not, is asking to be rejected. "I know one girl who plays a dizzy, dumb, cute brunette," a college student told me, waxing quite bitter about college women he calls "terminally cute." "Then when she gets drunk she exhibits a devastating wit. She's not as dumb as she appears."

What are the symptoms of being too cute? "Wearing lots of cute things—lots of pink, or pink and white ribbons in their hair, pony tails every day of the week. 'Hi, I wear pink all the time and I carry three teddy bears wherever I go.' That's a real worry at my school. Some girls' rooms have 18 teddy bears on the wall, and they give them individual names and talk to them while you're there. Yecch!"

Nancy tries too hard in a different way, by aquiescing too easily to a man's demands. She is a pretty woman, with soft, curly blonde hair, but she is too eager, too willing, to do exactly what a man wishes her to do. As her friend, Ted, told me, "The trouble with Nancy is that she is so darned available. She will do anything I want, any time I want . . . if I don't call her for a month, she's still eager to see me, and she's let me know that she's always there sexually and in every other way no matter what I do or how I treat her. That makes me nervous. I would like to be in love with Nancy because she does have some fine qualities, but I can't bring myself to say the words. I just can't make myself. Something about her turns me off, that's all."

A particularly pathetic type is the woman who is too eager to get married. "I danced with this woman one week," relates Peter. "We danced a couple of dances—she came up and asked me—and the next week I showed up at the dance and she came up to me and put her arms around me and told me she loved me. And I said, 'Now, wait a minute . . . !' And that's not the only instance of that I've seen. There is this one woman in [my] singles group, you really have to watch out for her. You have three dates with her and she wants to marry you."

Putting Up Barriers. Some women *say* they want to be sexy, but their actions speak otherwise, putting up a barrier between them and the very men they would attract. Men sense women who are putting up a wall and react against it. Here are some samples of barriers that men gave me:

* Not flirting
* Acting like men (acting tough)
* Showing lack of interest in men
* Having abrasive personality
* Having prima donna personality
* Being too critical or pessimistic
* Not liking men
* Being stuck-up
* Seeming not to have *real* feelings
* Displaying cranky or indifferent expression

The most negative thing a woman can do is complain, one man insisted. "It drags you down. Suppose two women are sitting in a bar and both are equally attractive. One of them says, 'Gee, this piano player is the worst one I've ever heard,' and the other one says, 'Hey, I really like that music.' Which one do you think is going to be considered sexier?"

"Whining!" echoed Ken, a systems analyst. "I guess that's my one big pet peeve about what women do to turn me off. Talking about all the bad things their husband did to them, over and over and over, it can be a real downer, it can turn your whole mood down. I mean, I know some people are really bitter and they need this, they have to let it out. But I feel like saying to them, 'Look, come back in six months when things are better again.'"

Bets is a good example of a whiner. Bets goes on a date with a man armed with a long list of complaints, on everything from the way her children treat her, to a fight she is having with a car dealership over the "lemon" of a car she bought. Bets even entertains her dates with stories of other·men she has gone out with, their bad habits, and the ways in which they have offended her. Her litany is, "The world is full of frogs—there aren't any princes." Certainly Bets has a hard time getting men to take her out more than once, and she seldom receives compliments that she is sexy.

Bad Habits.   There are some personal habits or vices, unfortunately, that turn men off very quickly—at least, the men who don't have that particular habit themselves. Here are some, named by men:

- Smoking
- Drinking
- Being drunk
- Chewing fingernails
- Chewing and popping gum
- Being a "druggie"

In this era of militant nonsmokers, many men find smoking in a woman to be an automatic turn-off, and nonsmoking men frequently will reject a woman for that without a second thought. Wayne is a nonsmoker who actually airs his clothing in the garage after having been in a smoke-filled atmosphere. "I won't ever date a smoker," he says emphatically. "I hate the smell of smoke in my clothes and in my hair—you can smell it the next day if you've been in a smoky bar—and I certainly wouldn't want to be with a woman who smoked."

Many men mentioned alcoholic behavior, in its various forms, as a real negative. "A turn-off to me is when a woman's eyes are sunken and they lack sparkle," one man said plainly. "A drinking problem causes this, which is in itself a giant turn-off. A woman into alcohol is not into men but into herself."

Gloria is engaged in a love affair with alcohol, a factor that robs her of sex appeal and turns her into a pathetic and lonely creature. When Gloria is feeling good, she's an attractive, well-dressed lady who attracts male attention. But male eyes quickly glaze when Gloria downs her fourth—and fifth—glass of wine.

One New Years' Eve, Gloria arrived at a party, and on her way into the parking lot, accidentally smashed a man's fender. Later, she walked around the party with the stiff-yet-wobbly look of the drunk. By 11:30 PM she was slumped at a table with her head in her hands.

"I avoid alcoholics like the plague," Don told me. He was one of the men Gloria had tried to approach. "I went with one once. Now if I even suspect that a woman might have problems with the bottle, I'm gone, just like that. I don't think it's sexy, I don't think it's attractive at all, it's just a total turn-off to me."

Poor Choices.   In seeking to be sexy, some women go overboard in choosing clothes or jewelry, and this sends a negative message to certain men. Men tend to want things in moderation, and will bristle at extremes. For example, men named these as choices that turned them off:

- Large print or plaid clothes
- Too much make-up
- Too-red lipstick
- Hair spray
- Long earrings
- Wild-looking clothes
- Designer jeans on women too broad in the beam
- Bad teeth

- Hair on upper lip
- Too much eye shadow
- Too much perfume

In some cases, a woman tolerates some minor flaw in herself that—with the help of a good doctor or dentist—could be fixed. Carrie detracts from her sexiness by not getting her teeth fixed. A tall, blonde woman of 35, Carrie has alabaster skin, big blue eyes, and a nice figure. But as soon as Carrie smiles, her assets go bankrupt. Not only does she have a back tooth missing, but she also has a sizeable space between her front teeth.

One cap and an inexpensive session with dental bonding would fix Carrie's smile. Why hasn't she taken that step? Instead of receiving sexy vibes, men are distracted by the gap in Carrie's teeth and are asking themselves why she doesn't go to the dentist.

Naomi is another woman who allows a fixable flaw to interfere with her sex appeal. Naomi has a medium-sized, hairy mole on her upper lip—a mole that could be removed by a dermatologist in a fifteen-minute procedure. Has Naomi grown so accustomed to the mole that she doesn't see it anymore? Possibly. But by ignoring her mole she is also robbing herself of that extra little fillip of sexiness.

Acting Low Class or Cheap.   Whether we can all agree on what behavior is "cheap" or "trashy," men have their own opinions, and woe to the woman who comes across to them as brassy or crude. As one woman pointed out to me, what you dress to attract is usually what you get. Here are behaviors that men named as turn-offs to them:

- Loudness
- Poor grammar
- Cheap looks
- Loud, abrasive voice
- Poor voice patterns
- Crude actions
- Swearing
- Bad manners

- Yelling
- Low class body action
- Flirting with too many men
- Talking too much about sex

One man admitted to me that some of his turn-offs were probably cultural. "But cheap, loud, trashy, vulgar, *my* interpretations—are turn-offs to me."

Said one sexy woman, "I know this woman with fingernails as long as daggers. She's a very heavy, bleached blonde with super tight pants—to men that will either be a turn-off, or they'll be out for only one thing. That's what she's showing she wants."

Provocative behavior is a powerful sexual weapon when used with discretion, but it can also be carried too far and be considered a turn-off. Men love provocative clothing, when they feel it is directed toward them alone. But if they feel that the clothes are being used as a sexual sweep—to gather up just any man—then they quickly lose interest.

Peg is an example of a woman who dresses too blatantly for the occasion. Peg apparently thinks that being sexy means attiring herself as if it were New Year's Eve. When the other women are wearing casual dresses or jumpsuits, Peg shows up in a slinky black evening dress with spaghetti straps and a neckline that plunges down between her breasts. A slit on her thigh nearly reveals the tops of her panty hose. Peg's make-up is extreme, too, with dark dollops of rouge on her cheeks. In her hair she has sprayed silver glitter.

What Peg doesn't appear to realize is that her clothes are sending out this strong message: *I'll have sex with almost anyone.* She is advertising herself as being nonselective. On several occasions I noticed Peg in this gear, standing near the bar being eyed by men. Yes, some men did approach her. But for every man who talked to her, there were dozens of others who glanced at her and stayed away.

"You can tell what she's out for," one man told me, looking at Peg from across the room. "One-night stands and penicillin city. I wouldn't be caught dead being seen with that. Just looking at her gives me the creepy-crawlies."

Commented another man that same night: "She wouldn't dress the way she does if she wasn't looking to be noticed. I tend to be very leery of someone who would go too far with that. A little bit goes a long way. If you put too many of those factors together, it's questionable whether I'd want to be involved. I'd conclude that that person is involved with too many people."

Personality Flaws.   Here is an area that a woman might not be able to change much—but men do take note of personality defects, and when they spot them, they are immediately repelled. Here are some samples men gave me:

- Lack of intelligence
- Complains
- No sense of humor
- Negative attitudes
- No zest or energy
- Self-centered attitude
- Dishonesty
- Jealousy
- Bitter attitude
- Anger
- Looking for a free ride
- Materialistic
- Clinging vine

Despite Madonna's song, *Material Girl,* materialism, or any hint of it, is a quick dash in the face of sex appeal. And apparently a number of women are so financially needy that they come on like bankers taking a man's monetary measure. "I've had women on the dance floor bluntly ask me what I do and how much money I make. When I told one woman that I worked for Detroit Edison," said one man, "She turned around and left me right there on the dance floor, just walked away. Too many women think of sex as a commodity to be meted out, and that is a real turn-off."

But one of the biggest personality handicaps—a far greater handicap than any amount of fat—is bitterness. A woman can have a gorgeous face and body, and ruin it all by the poison of bitterness. Margie is 36 and her petite, nicely-proportioned figure gains her a lot of second looks from men. However, two bad marriages and several failed relationships have left Margie with a legacy of anger, bubbling so near the surface that it frequently breaks through.

Margie complains that "there aren't any good men," bitterly saying that "the men all want younger women." When she attends social functions there is an angry look on her face, and her body language is angry, too.

A happy ending to this story, though: two months ago Margie joined a therapy group for women in transition, and is beginning to work through some of her bitterness with the help of the group. "I guess I do send out negative messages," she admitted. "But I'm starting to get past that, I'm starting to see where my anger *really* belongs, and it's a good feeling. I don't have to talk about it so much anymore. And yesterday, I got a phone call from a man I'd met at work, inviting me to go out to dinner. He told me that I was the prettiest woman in the office!"

Axioms of Sex Appeal

1. A big turn-on for a man is *confidence*. Men repeatedly told me that. If a woman lacks a perfect body, her self-esteem, her body confidence, will make her seem sexy anyway.

2. Men are also attracted when a woman shows strong interest in them—without overdoing it.

3. Turn-offs to men are as varied as are men, and many of them are idiosyncratic, but there are enough common male dislikes to be worth listening to. Many turn-offs read like a list of the things our mothers taught us *never* to do—yet apparently thousands of women are doing them.

4. There are some sins a woman commits that say, loudly and clearly, that she doesn't consider herself sexy and doesn't care to try. These include slovenliness, dirtiness, and body odor.

5. Some turn-offs fall into the area of poor self-esteem. The woman doesn't feel good about herself, and she projects this attitude by having bad posture, being sloppy overweight, having a lack of muscle tone, and lack of confidence.

6. Some women try too hard, and their very desperateness turns men off. Being too aggressive, too needy, too "cute," or too materialistic will drive men away very quickly.

7. Another turn-off happens unconsciously when women put up barriers to being sexy, such as being too critical or pessimistic, acting too male, being abrasive, stuck-up, or indifferent.

8. Bad habits are a huge turn-off, and many men said that the two biggest turn-offs to them are smoking and alcoholic behavior.

9. Using too much of anything is usually a turn-off to men. Poor choices in clothes, jewelry, or perfume send out negative rather than positive vibes. Also, sometimes a woman tolerates some minor flaw in herself that could be fixed with the aid of a good dentist or dermatologist. Bad teeth and facial moles or hair definitely detract from sex appeal.

10. Acting what men consider "low class" or "cheap" is another quick turn-off, and men tend to resent loud, abrasive voices, women's acting crude, swearing, using "low class body action," or dressing too provocatively.

11. Personality flaws—some of which can't be helped—can nonetheless dampen sexual attractiveness. One of the greatest defects is bitterness, which handicaps a woman far greater than any amount of fat.

11

Sexiness in Our Lives

Don't ever tell me that having large breasts is fun. When I was 15 I couldn't walk down the hallway without boys whistling and making comments, it happened 6 times a day. Even my sister cuttingly told me that I was built exactly like Jayne Mansfield. I started slumping to hide myself. To this day I have these terrible mixed feelings about my breasts . . .

—Female interviewee

Reactions to the very-sexy woman can range from the amusing to the obsessive. One English musical director found the legendary Brigitte Bardot more than just a little exciting. Working on a television special with the sex goddess, he couldn't take his eyes off her. That day, Bardot was wearing a very-short mini, and her legs were perfectly, alluringly tanned.

Said one observer: "This poor bloke was obsessed! He followed her everywhere, his eyes glued to her legs. If she changed seats, he'd suddenly be sitting in the chair opposite her. It was getting just a little bit embarrassing, I must admit."

The Englishman's visual surveillance continued the rest of the afternoon. Finally, Bardot reacted. She marched across the room to within a foot of the man's passion-flushed face, lifted her skirt daringly high, and snapped, "If that is all you want to see, you might as well have a good look."[1]

Most sexy women have experienced similar incidents, although not all react as snappily as Bardot. "One time I made the mistake of attending a "Shipwreck" singles party wearing a pair of short shorts," one woman told me. "I must admit it was an effective costume—in fact, another woman who saw me actually left the party and went home to change into her shorts, too. But the behavior of the men that night. . . . one man actually pinched me on the rear end. It was as if the shorts gave him the license to crawl all over me."

Ladies Home Journal's survey of 102,000 readers probed into women's feelings about themselves and their daily lives. As I mentioned in an earlier chapter, the magazine learned that of women who view themselves as "traditional," 46.4 percent considered themselves to be sexy, while 64.3 percent of women who think of themselves as "new women," feel sexy.[2]

However, sex appeal, for many women, is a mixed bag. There are times when owning it is an enormous pleasure, other times women feel they must downplay that part of themselves, put their sexiness "on hold." Many women have anxieties, even anger, about sex appeal. If they feel they haven't got enough of it, they may feel resentment toward other women they perceive as having "more."

Said one very attractive woman in her late 30s: "Yes, I've been told by men that I'm sexy to the point that I've had to accept that as a part of myself, even though it has been hard at times. I mean, what is it about me that has that effect on people? It has always startled me that men, once even a man who came to the door selling funeral plots, have come on to me as a sexy woman. Men I've had relationships with have told me that I'm unusually sexy, and that they respond to me with much more sexual force than to other women, especially in bed. 'I don't know what it is about you,' they say. *I* don't know what it is either. I'm just me. I don't act provocative. But I come across that way."

Of the women I polled, the majority said that they feel they are not doing anything special to be sexy. Others said they try hard to be as sexually appealing as they can. Smaller numbers of women admitted to more negative feelings: "It makes me feel puzzled sometimes: I wonder, why me?" "I feel guilty sometimes because I have what others don't." "I sometimes wish I could turn off this quality I have." "I feel angry sometimes because other women seem to be sexier than I am." "I don't feel very sexy at all." "Sometimes the aggravation of being sexy isn't worth what I get from it."

Nancy C. Baker, author of *The Beauty Trap,* writes, "Physical appearance is so important, in one sense, and so unimportant, in another, that it's not surprising that most of us experience ambivalent feelings about it. The truth is, our entire society is ambivalent about beauty. We can't decide whether beauty is good or evil, powerful or weak, an advantage or a disadvantage, safe or dangerous."[3]

Baker tells about being a teenaged car hop in the 60s, when the boys "came to the drive-in to get their kicks from harrassing me. 'Hey, Blondie, what time you gettin' off tonight?' one might shout at me. Another might yank my ponytail or my apron strings as I turned away. A third might offer a shrill wolf whistle. . . . "[4]

Baker recalls having felt a mixed bag of emotions at this treatment. Sometimes it was flattery—after all, she was getting more wolf whistles than the other car hops. Still, there was also embarrassment, anger, and fear. "There was also the remote possibility that one of those boys might be waiting in the dark. I don't remember articulating my exact fear at the time, but it was of rape."

"There was another emotion I felt, too. . . . that emotion was guilt. A little of the guilt was over my feeling flattered. In addition, I felt that there must be something about the way I looked or talked or tilted my head that *caused* these boys to act in a very disrespectful way. Perhaps their behavior was *my* fault, not theirs. I felt ashamed."[5]

When I asked the women I surveyed to note what advice they would give to a daughter about sex appeal, nearly all marked two items: "Achieve on your own merits, don't depend on being sexy," and "Enjoy your own sexuality as a woman." But the third most frequently marked statement (more than 50 percent) was "Be careful that you don't allow men to use you." One third of the women marked "Being sexy is not always a blessing."

Downplaying their sex appeal is a reality in the lives of most sexy women, at least occasionally. Usually it's done for four reasons: To avoid attracting the wrong man, to avoid offending a lover, to save the feelings of other women, and to avoid hassles at work.

"When do I turn off my sex appeal? When someone's coming on stronger than I want them to," was a typical answer. One woman told me about downplaying her sexuality as a teenager in front of her father.

Said another, "Sometimes I don't go out without attracting about eleven guys. The only time I turn it off is when I see that I'm hurting someone else by it. I have a girlfriend with a hooked nose, she had two or three operations on it but it didn't get much better, and she's got black, frizzy hair. I'll go out with her, but sometimes she feels terrible. I dress down when I'm with her."

In their work life is when many women find sex appeal a disadvantage. More than half of the women said that they downplay their sexual attractiveness because it would not be appropriate at work. Twenty-seven said they have learned to deal with sexual attentions by being cool and businesslike on the job, and many said they deliberately select low-key business wear that does not emphasize their figure.

These actions are apparently quite necessary. Sexuality has entered the workplace, and in corporations across the land, wherever men and women are working together, sexual excitement has added spice and adventure to the humdrum office routine. Love affairs between co-workers, or between worker and boss, are growing more common, and where once women complained about sexual harrassment, growing numbers of women are now *seeking* some kind of sexual excitement at work.

According to a headline for one article in *Cosmopolitan, "Today's office smoulders with erotic heat. Affairs are everywhere, questions too. Like who (if anyone) is off limits?"* Phrases from the article read like something from *True Confessions.* "Sex is on people's minds at work . . . in the cafeteria of a major hospital or a huge manufacturing outfit, you'll see a flirty crowd of potential lovers. . . . Much of the rampant sexual energy of the workplace is harmless stuff. People like to feel attractive and they like to be turned on. . . . For those involved in real affairs, however, the office scene is supercharged. . . . "[6]

According to a *Penthouse* survey, 84 percent of the men said they have been propositioned by a female co-worker at one time or another, and 70 percent took the women up on their offer.[7]

What is life like for a sexy woman at work? Some of the women pointed out to me that they don't work around men, so sex doesn't enter into the workplace for them. But two-thirds of the women said that they received compliments on their looks, body, etc., from male co-workers. More than half said men often flirted with them on the job. One-quarter said that married men approached them, and of the 60, 12 had had an affair with men they worked with.

One-fourth of the women said that they have experienced sexual harrassment on the job; 5 said they had to avoid going to certain areas in their workplace because of the male attention they would receive there. Five women said they had to change jobs because of sexual harrassment, and one said she feared rape from a man she worked with.

Women working blue-collar jobs are usually subject to the grosser expressions of sexual harrassment. "Only a few years ago in the factory where I work, all the women who work on trim were expected to put out sexually for any manager that wanted them," Cindy told me.

Cindy works afternoons at an automobile plant, a job that puts her in contact with a lot of men who harrass her in every way from wolf whistles to suggestive language to out-and-out propositions. One man was fired from his job for harassing several women, including Cindy. To her consternation, about a year later the union managed to get him his job back.

"Somebody told me he was back, and I thought they were kidding, but that night I saw him and I thought I would die. He had been really something before—he had actually pushed me up against a wall. I handled it, though. I just avoided contact with him. I avoided eye contact, and I acted as if he was not even there. It's easy to do that—you don't show a response, or any fear, you completely ignore them, you pretend you don't even hear what they say."

White-collar women receive a more subtle kind of harrassment. "Last month I was approached at the water cooler by this married guy," said one woman, an office manager. "He started asking me if I'd like to come out and have a drink with him. 'What?' I said. I was playing kind of dumb. He said, 'Would you like to have a drink with me? You single women must be kind of deprived.' I really almost laughed out loud. I told him, 'The only ones who are deprived are the married men who are asking single women for dates.'"

A man told me about a sexy woman who works in the same building he does, as a receptionist. She is 24 and vaguely resembles a Playboy bunny. "Married men have been hitting on Kimmie ever since she has been here. One supervisor let her drive his motorcycle during the lunch hour—well, it wasn't exactly lunch time and he had no business doing that. She crashed the bike on company property and bruised her arm. He realized that he was a jackass, playing with his job. She could have sued—she had an accident on company property on *his* bike . . . She still doesn't realize he's hitting on her, she thinks he's just being nice to her."

"I'm in sales and my sexuality can be a big problem some-times," one brunette, with clear, exquisite skin, related to me. "It's the old story, they think that I come right along with the product. It's a fine line, I have to sell myself as a person, and yet keep my sexuality played down."

Professor Sandra Harley Cooley, sociologist at the University of Texas at San Antonio, surveyed 481 working women on the type of harrassment they had experienced. All of them said they had experienced something. Sixteen percent said the advances were so disturbing they resigned, while 36 percent said they were subjected to leering or ogling, and 37 percent complained of hints or verbal pressures. Eighteen percent were asked away for a weekend by male supervisors, 6 percent were promised rewards for sex, and 3 percent were subjected to touching, grabbing, pinching, or fondling.[8]

Often the male view of harrassment is that this doesn't occur without some encouragement. A quote from one male corporate executive: "Women should be aware that they are judged by what they wear and what they talk about. If they wear suggestive clothing they are asking for it. Also a sexy women won't be taken seriously in business."

Unfortunately, the boundaries of sexual harrassment are being blurred considerably by the phenomenon of sex that is currently sweeping the workplace. When sex is an added fillip of excitement, changing work from dull to dynamite, the boundaries become unclear. Who wants a man to approach her, and who doesn't? Will the woman welcome a flirtation? These days, many do.

Underneath their subdued business garb, many business women are wearing frilly and sexy lingerie, apparently in an effort to feel their femininity despite the restrictions of the office. Said one corporate business woman: "Sometimes I think of myself as a wonderful surprise package. . . . There's the way I seem to be on the outside. But there's the way I could be if someone dared untie me. . . . "

A telling anecdote appears in Liz Roman Gallese's book, *Women Like Us: What Is Happening to the Women of the Harvard Business School Class of '75*. "Mary Pat," one of the female class members, once dressed up as a Playboy bunny at a Halloween party and danced on a table top. On another occasion, she campaigned for office wearing a blonde wig, gold lame boots, and purple-velvet hot pants.

Says author Gallese: "Mary Pat seemed to symbolize what women have to deny for the sake of access to the alien world of business. The asexual female executive was crying out to be recognized for the sexual woman she really was."[9]

In the social world, sexuality becomes even more confusing. Although numbers of the women I surveyed were divorced, most were in steady relationships. Others were married. Still, the picture of what happens to a sexy women in a social framework is an interesting one. One woman told me that a man "came on" to her and invited her to go on a cruise with him at a party she and her husband were giving, with her husband only fifteen feet away in the kitchen!

Some of the women I surveyed checked off nearly all of the 16 items on my questionaire that covered social situations. Nearly all said that, in social settings, men openly compliment their looks or their body. Two-thirds of the women said that men often flirt with them, and that they receive friendly kisses and hugs from men they are not dating.

Apparently these women do exert a strong attraction over men in general, for more than one-third of the respondents said that men "get crushes" on them, and even men they encounter casually start showing signs of coming on to them. Two-thirds said that men who are much younger, or much older than they are, show signs of being very attracted to them. Twenty-three women said that a man they associate with socially has made it clear that he has feelings of love for them.

"I got myself in trouble flirting one night," Betti, 39, admitted. "I thought, 'Oh, my God, I shouldn't do this.' The man was really, really responding, but he was too new and too raw for me to be doing this, I really overdid it. He was the kind of person you could really flirt with—so much fun I couldn't resist. Then suddenly he just started shaking. I had gotten too far past the point where he couldn't resist."

Tracey, 34, often generates unrest on the social scene. Tracey, who dates a male friend of mine, is tall and auburn-haired, with the saucy, pouty, high-cheekboned look of the centerfold. Sex appeal oozes from her, even in the candid photograph I saw of her in a family setting.

Taking Tracey to a nightclub or bar-lounge is not always a simple project, my friend tells me. Other men somehow start closing in, moving closer and closer and even striking up conversations with Tracey. If she leaves to go to the restroom, men excuse themselves and lie in wait for her by the door to the women's room.

"I've almost gotten into fights several times because of this," says Ken. "And I've ended up taking Tracey and getting out of there. Everywhere I take her, the men are turning on to her, and she says she isn't doing anything to cause it." He seems almost pleased and proud. "But you have to admit, she is awfully sexy, darn it."

Jan told me about a date she had to go dancing that turned awkward when her date left to go to the restroom. "Suddenly I looked up and there was this guy standing by the booth where I was sitting, leaning in and staring at me. He just point-blank asked me if I would like to go home with him that night.

"I told him no and asked him to leave—and he wouldn't. That really scared me. Here was this drunk leaning into the booth and blocking my way. Finally I stood up and pushed my way past him. I went and waited outside the door of the men's room for my date to come out, and we left right away. I could tell that my date wasn't very pleased and I didn't blame him— but it wasn't my fault."

Harrassment is part of the social picture, for many. Twenty-five women answered yes to the statement that, "men have deliberately touched my body (patted me, stroked me) at parties," while 15 said that "men whistle or make suggestive comments about me within my hearing." Twenty women admitted that a man had "made himself unpleasantly persistent," while 13 said they have experienced sexual harrassment from a man at a party, club meeting, or social event. Eight feared rape from a man they were dating or encountered socially, and 1 actually was raped.

Kerry, a woman with a voluptuous D-cup figure, told me about an incident at a party. "Someone was taking pictures, and he started out by making remarks about how I should stand right in front of the camera so my profile would stand out. Then he 'accidentally' brushed up against my breasts. When I pulled back, he very sarcastically said he was 'sorry,' in a way that told me he had done it on purpose. I was angry, but I'm not the type to create a fuss. So what I did was go sit down in the middle of a group of about 8 women, and start giving them a description of what he had done. We were still talking about it when the man himself came up to our group and sat down. I didn't lower my voice or stop telling the story, so he had to sit there and listen to the truth. All the women were listening, and he had made a total fool of himself."

"Most sexual harrassment is because of the crudity and lack of class of the men," another woman told me. "I remember I was dancing with a man, and he said, 'Wait until you see what's in my pants.' That'll be the day."

Diana Warshay, a sociology professor at Wayne State University, Detroit, has been studying catcalls, wolf whistles and suggestive comments that occur when a woman passes a group of men. One-third of the women I interviewed said they are regularly catcalled, either at work or in social situations.

As Warshay has pointed out women are seen as good or bad. They are to be either protected or disrespected. A man is the protector, and a good woman isn't supposed to go anyplace alone. If a woman is attached to a man, then another man would have to challenge him. That's why a woman who is walking with a man is not bothered.

Dr. Warshay adds that the catcall phenomenon isn't limited to our culture, but occurs all over the world, more prevalent in big cities than small towns, because the more anonymity the catcaller has, the less bound by social controls he feels. It also happens more when the men are in groups.

One man was quoted as saying that he considered his cat-calling activities "flirting." "How did I know she liked it? I'd see a smile sometimes. If she smiles and says 'no thanks,' you try again. But if she turns her head or pretends not to hear, you keep moving."

Warshay says there is some controversy over whether or not a woman should talk back to these street Romeos. Much harrassment has to do with body language, she adds. The woman who walks in a lackadaisical manner, dawdling down the street, gives the impression she can be victimized. The best thing is to walk as if you mean business, with a purposeful stride and your head up.

Being Beautiful

"My looks are just average," said one 33-year-old female executive rather pathetically. "I have wanted to be different all my life. I envy the tall, slim, glamorous woman. Every time I look in the mirror and see my unglamorous face and figure, I could cry."

For those of us born average looking, the world of the super-beautiful is one filled with envy and a lot of fantasies that we create in our own minds. But is being beautiful the carefree, idealized life we visualize it to be?

As most women suspect, the life of a beautiful woman definitely *is* different, and this difference starts right at birth. Suppose two little girls are born, and one is what adults consider a beauty, a fetching infant that people *oooh* over and fathers pay extra attention to. But the other baby . . . well, she's average looking.

Will the girls be treated differently as they grow up? Yes, says Dr. Judith Langlois, a developmental psychologist at the University of Texas at Austin, who has studied the effects of physical appearance on children.

Pretty babies get more parental attention right from birth. Mothers tend to nuzzle and kiss exceptionally pretty babies more often, and seem to be more involved with them, better able to predict and meet their needs than the mothers of unattractive infants, Langlois has learned. Fathers of these appealing infants expect to spend more time taking care of them, and actually *do* put in more time at fathering.

The extra attention continues. On the first day of school, the pretty child's cute appearance will set off an unconscious expectation in her teacher, says Langlois, who talked about two hypothetical children, beautiful Jennifer, and plainer Lily.

"The teacher will assume that Jennifer is bright, well adjusted, popular, and well behaved. She'll expect Jennifer to do well in classwork, share her toys, and help other children. Lily's appearance will set off just the opposite set of expectations."[10]

As the girls grow up, Jennifer will be what Langlois calls a "sociometric star," that is, lots of kids in her class will like her, and many children will want to be her friend. The plainer Lily will have best friends, too—but she might not get her choice. The most beautiful girls in her class will probably not choose her to be her best friend.

Beautiful little girls become the focus of adult adulation or even demands. There is a whole system of beauty contests for children, for instance, and the competition is fierce, replete with rivalries and tears. "She's always been the center of attention," says the mother of a 7-year-old contestant in the "Missy Miss" division of a children's beauty contest. "Adults are very awed by her."[11]

Cybill Shepherd talks about beautiful children and the attention they receive. "People lay trips on beautiful women," she told *McCalls.* "Men tell my daughter that she's a 'killer.' And I say, 'What do you *mean?*' They say, 'She's going to break a lot of hearts.' Now what kind of thing is that for a six-year-old kid to hear? It's the way people think about beautiful women—that they're killers, vamps out to destroy people's lives—it's that negative."[12]

As the exceptionally pretty woman grows up, she finds herself automatically considered to have certain good qualities, such as honesty, warmth, intelligence—far more of these qualities than her plainer sisters. And yet, other studies have shown that when a beautiful women is trying to succeed in business, people will take her less seriously.

Letty Cottin Pogrebin mentions the "beauty tyrannies" imposed on women. For the super-beautiful, there is the built-in obsolescence of aging. For minority women, it is being pressured to meet standards set by the white majority. For moderately attractive women, it is the suffering of "not feeling beautiful enough," and for plain women, it is the fear of being unlovable and unloved.[13]

Being regarded only for your looks can be a scary experience. Although I am certainly not beautiful, I remember an occasion a few years ago when my ex-husband and I made a trip to England, and became friends with another couple, who we met on the plane. I was astonished when the other man, Rod, kept complimenting me, telling me how attractive I was. He even told me that I would fit in very well in his office, where "we hire gals with looks, and an ugly girl just wouldn't fit in."

The compliments were nice, but the more time we spent with Rod and Sarah, the more uneasy I became. Rod kept emphasizing that beauty was all-important—that a woman didn't exist for him unless she had fantastic looks. It occurred to me that Rod could care less about *me*. It was my looks that drew him. It was a curiously dehumanizing experience; in fact, it was deep-down scary. Years later, when I became divorced, I remembered Rod. When I attended singles groups I carefully wore my eyeglasses, so that I would scare off all the Rods, and attract a type of man who wanted me for *me*.

Looks

Sometimes looks narrow a woman's horizons or compromise her personal freedom. I lived briefly in Hawaii, which is overloaded with nubile young females who parade their bodies on the beaches. Even in that setting, Linn, 20, was a knockout. With her shapely body and mane of white-blonde hair, she looked like a very innocent yet alluring centerfold. She was also newly married, jobless, and stuck at home all day in a small, isolated cottage on Maui.

It sounds ideal, doesn't it? Beautiful girl, beautiful island, time to explore. But life for Linn was curiously restricting. There was a wild beach a half-mile away from where Linn lived, and Linn longed to go there to sunbathe and snorkel. However, the beach was unsupervised, and going there alone meant for Linn a constant succession of male heckling and approaches, even possible danger of rape. Other young women, mind you, could and did go to the very same beach without harm. But they didn't look like Linn.

Several times Linn did make the trek through the woods to the beach, only to be harrassed and to leave in fear. Finally she gave up. Her sexy looks limited the places she could go and the wild beach was off limits to her.

Many beautiful women get turned into objects or possessions, prized by men who want someone they can show off to other men. Men who will date only beautiful women have been called *beauty junkies.* These men are tellingly described in this sentence from *Worldly Goods,* by Michael Korda: "In the end, all they wanted was a woman who could make other men envious of them—somebody to show off at parties as living proof that they were still in the game, winners in bed as well as in business."[14]

Beauty junkies attack a woman's self-esteem. Said one attractive dancer angrily, "He's saying that beauty is the most important thing about a woman—that's insult number one. Insult number two is . . . most of us can never measure up. In other words, if there were only one woman in the world prettier than I, he'd choose her. How can we not feel like second choice? How can we help but feel insecure? We're always in danger of being rejected."

Another woman tells about a New Year's Eve, when her boyfriend asked her to wear a low-cut, red, slinky dress with rows and rows of jiggly, suggestive fringe. "Part of me felt terrific," she told *Mademoiselle.* "I knew what he meant. It was a very sexy, flattering outfit. . . . To be honest, though, I got real upset. People would be ogling me. I was self-conscious—that's why I'd never worn that thing out in public before! Mainly, I didn't think my boyfriend cared how I looked. He was asking me to dress up to make *him* look good. I resented that . . . a lot!"[15]

Carrying beauty one step further and adding exceptional sex appeal, then mixing with Hollywood, can create a sex goddess. With sex goddess status comes a whole new set of problems. When Raquel Welch first came to Hollywood, for example, she was bombarded by unwanted male attention. Men harassed her, even waiting around in front of her building for her to appear. Said Raquel, "These are the men who won't take no for an answer. You can't get rid of them. . . . If you didn't answer the phone or the doorbell they'd find something to bash through the glass. I was always moving with my kids in the dark of the night. I found that men can be pretty tough."[16]

Women who have been touted as sex goddesses often find they are playing the role that society has set up for them, stifling private bitterness.

Raquel Welch, for example, has played the part of quintessential sex object for a whole generation of men, who have even incorporated her name into their language, using it to *stand* for sex appeal. I once received a compliment from a lover: "I'd walk over Raquel Welch to get to you."

What does Raquel think about this dehumanizing, this manufacturing of herself into a celluloid, not-quite-real image?

"People sit and wait for me to turn them on," she has said. "I think to myself, what the hell, why should I come on to some guy? It's not *me* he's especially interested in. It's Raquel Welch! The label. He's after the label. To have it said that you're a sex symbol, the most beautiful girl in the world, is initially terrific. You think, isn't that neat? . . . Nobody can be the most beautiful girl in the world. It's just fairytale time. There was a huge discrepancy between the symbol—Raquel Welch—and what I could ever aspire to be for real. The stupidity of it is that once somebody says you're something, you try to *be* it."[17]

"You know," she told *Rolling Stone,* "When people meet me they usually change their minds about me. But I can't meet everyone. Do you know when my English hairdresser told friends she was coming to work with me they told her: 'That old bitch surrounds herself with a lot of trolls. She can't bear to have beautiful women anywhere near.' Isn't that an incredible thing to say about someone you don't even know? I know I'm supposed to be a sex symbol, but the truth is I'm not a terribly sexy person. Not unless I'm emotionally involved with a man. Then it's different. So I suppose I disappoint a lot of people when they meet me. They've read about this great sex symbol and they expect extraordinary things of me. But what can I do? I mean, I can't just stand there undulating, can I?"[18]

Three months before she died, Marilyn Monroe told Peter Levathes, the head of the studio at Twentieth Century Fox: "I'm a failure as a woman. My men expect so much of me, because of the image they've made of me and that I've made of myself, as a sex symbol. Men expect so much, and I can't live up to it. They expect bells to ring and whistles to whistle, but my anatomy is the same as any other woman's. I can't live up to it."[19]

And even Dustin Hoffman, during his sojourn into the streets of New York dressed as a woman for his role as *Tootsie,* said emphatically, "I *don't* like being a sex object. I find that unappealing and I understand why women don't like it—because it's not good for your ego. You're replaceable."

Some sex goddesses come to believe their own screen image, playing the role that Hollywood has laid out for them. Jayne Mansfield, for instance, played to the hilt her goddess role. Writes Martha Saxton in her book, *Jayne Mansfield and the American Fifties,* "Jayne suffered from the sexual stereotype forced on a woman with a forty-inch bust. There was nothing else she could be but sexy, and there was no way anyone could respond to her but sexually."

Like many women who have been strikingly beautiful all their lives, Mansfield counted on men to provide her with a high level of energy and electricity, and knew men only in relation to her sexuality. Saxton writes, "She had never developed any tools for finding out much about people, so when she'd exhausted the sex, she'd exhausted the relationship."[20]

Mansfield at times grew discouraged and even afraid of her own powers. "I have never met a man who didn't make a pass at me," she said once. "They start by wanting to be my friend. The old ones are worse than the young ones. We talk a while and sooner or later I find that they are not listening to me. They just keep staring and moving closer."[21]

Mae West was another screen goddess who was preoccupied with the image of herself as a sex object. She interpreted any incident as a tribute to her allure. One time she proudly pointed out to a friend what she called the "Overcoat Brigade," men seated in the first couple of rows of her performances who were masturbating under their coats. Mae interpreted this as a great compliment. In one Connecticut town she had a dressing room on a courtyard, where local boys kept trying to peep in to see her undressed. "The more they peeked the more excited she got," said a friend.

In some screen sex symbols there is a strong tendency to exhibitionism—a factor I also noticed in several of the sexy women I interviewed for this book. One woman, noted at the singles group she attends for her flashy dancing style, kept saying things in her interview like, "I get the attention."

Dolly Parton told an interviewer about wanting to show off her body even as a schoolgirl. "I always wore tight clothes. When I walked down the hall, everybody was a-lookin' to see how tight my skirt was that day or how tight my sweater was.

I never did like to go around half naked but a lotta people said I might as well be naked, as tight as my clothes were. But even as a little bitty kid, if my Momma made me wear somethin' that was loose on me, I used to just *cry*. I wanted my clothes to fit me. Even though they was just rags, I wanted them to fit close to me."[22]

Sex symbols sometimes carry exhibitionism to its full, bizarre extreme. Marilyn Monroe, for instance, loved to show her body off to men and once gave a naked interview to publicist Joe Wohlander. Legends say that Marilyn disliked underwear and loathed wearing panties—and some candid photos published in *Hollywood Babylon* bear out this predilection.

Marilyn once flashed Mrs. Ben Bodney, wife of the owner of the Algonquin Hotel. Mrs. Bodney, walking along Fifth Avenue, happened to encounter Marilyn walking there, too, wearing a new mink coat. They stopped to chat, and when the wife of the hotelier asked what Marilyn was wearing with it, Marilyn responded, "Nothing," and snapped open her coat to prove it.

In 1955 Brigitte Bardot was shooting a film that required a nude scene, in an era where such daring scenes were shot by covering over the actress' pubic area and nipples, then photographing her through lace curtains or frosted glass. In this particular scene, Brigitte was supposed to take a shower behind a plastic curtain while Dirk Bogarde sat on the other side, getting hotter and hotter under the collar.

Unfortunately, no matter how much the crew adjusted the lights, the flannel over the actress' crotchline was still visible. Finally Brigitte screamed, *"Merde!"* peeled off the plaster and flannel panties, and stepped back into the shower. The scene was shot *au naturel*.

Plain Women

But what if we are not sex symbols? What if we are average looking or plain? Does that mean that we are automatically cut off from ever being considered sexy? Not according to the men I interviewed. I was pleased to learn that nearly one-fifth of the men thought a physically plain woman could be sexy "nearly always." More than half thought a plain woman could be sexy "sometimes." It's significant that *none* of the men said a plain woman could never be sexy.

There are actually advantages to being plain, if one chooses to search for them. Plain women don't have to worry about being victimized by beauty junkies. "I want men to be attracted to me for other reasons than just sexual attraction," one woman emphasized. Stated another, "If a man has the intelligence and sensitivity to look past my glasses, he's going to see a real person, the real me, and then he's worth meeting."

Ellen Seton wrote in *Mademoiselle* that a plain woman can capitalize on the asset of her secret vanities, the things she knows about herself that are fabulous, such as her soft, smooth skin, her appealingly full lips, or her perfect nose. Keeping a catalog of our positive assets is a real esteem-builder that adds to our inner sense of sex appeal.

There are two advantages that less-than-raving beauties have in their relationships. One is that men don't fall in love with them from afar, idealizing the relationship to the point where the woman can't live up to it. Instead men are "slowly smitten," rather than instantaneously, which works better in many love affairs anyway.

Second, stresses Seton, plain-looking women tend to have more realism in their romances. Too often, truly beautiful women suffer from a feeling of fraudulence—a fear that the man fell in love with them for what they look like, rather than for who they are. A more average-looking woman can feel secure that her lover wants her for *her,* not some myth that he carries around in his head.

Said Seton: "Even if the mirror proclaims us plain, an inner conviction that we are beautiful can make us so—or if not beautiful, decidedly attractive. And *attractive* is an interesting word. Although in usage it has come to mean the same things as *goodlooking,* it doesn't really refer to any objective physical attribute, but rather to a totally intangible force that can draw another person to us. We can't all be beautiful, but we can all be attractive. And that, I think, is the ultimate power."[23]

Need for a Man

When I first started writing this book I had a pet theory about sex appeal—that sexy women are partly sexy because they *need* a man in their lives more. Therefore, like a flower developing nectar in its blossoms to draw bees, they've developed those qualities that will draw men to them.

Perhaps to some extent this is true. Certainly some sex symbols have had extra-strong needs to have men around them. Jayne Mansfield, for instance, was a woman who couldn't live without male attention and approval, a woman for whom nothing was ever enough. She is quoted as saying, "With a figure like mine a girl is certain to attract attention, and I find it pleasing and *necessary* that a man look at me."[24] (Italics mine.)

Said Brigitte Bardot, "I must always have a new lover in sight before I am able to let the old one go. I must always be sure of one. So, of course, there is often this difficult time of change. I cannot live alone, you see. It is stupid but it is like that. I may be emancipated, but finally I am not free."[25]

But the more ordinary women I talked to exhibited a more middle-of-the-road attitude toward men. Yes, they need them— but not desperately. Most of the women I polled said they needed a man in their lives either "sometimes" or "usually," while only a few said they needed a man "nearly always." On the other hand, in response to the statement, *"I can get along without having a man around,"* nearly half said they "usually" can get along without him. Only 10 women, less than one-fifth, said they could get along without a man "nearly always."

"I have a real problem with the word 'need,' " said one woman. "That depends on the man. I'd rather have nobody than a jerk."

"I can survive without a man but I'm lots happier with one," Suzanne, 31, admitted to me. "It would be very, very hard for me to live alone and have no male friend or lover to see or be with. Male attention is important to me, and all the good things that go along with having a male around. I like the feeling that there is someone I can fall back on, depend on, even though I consider myself to be independent. I don't necessarily have to be married, but I want a man who is 'there' and who I can see nearly every day."

Wanting a man but being able to survive without one— perhaps it is this delicate balance that creates a sort of sensuous unrest that men find intriguing. One woman I interviewed, Terry, 39, is a classic example of a woman men consider sexy.

She receives as many as six telephone calls a day from men. Men flirt with her, ask her to lunch, try to have affairs with her, sexually harass her, get crushes on her, drop hints, make approaches. When she recently placed a singles ad, nearly every man she dated wanted to have a relationship with her.

One of Terry's secrets, I'm convinced, is her attitude toward needing a man in her life. Yes, Terry admits, she needs one. "There are times when I don't like being alone without a man in my life. That doesn't mean I have to have someone all the time. But I'm tired of being alone, tired of coming home to an empty place, tired of going to bed by myself. I don't like to think of the years ahead, living alone, and yet I fear commitment and making it successful."

Even in her statement to me, Terry expressed ambivalence. As much as she needs a man, she also distrusts them, and this dichotomy is, I think, what men sense. She wants them . . . but not too much. She needs them . . . but she can get along just fine by herself, thank you. This type of projected attitude is very comfortable and appealing to the man who is afraid of being clung to, who is terrified of a woman who is "looking for a meal ticket."

Other women expressed a yearning, a feeling of need—but again, always with a qualification. "I would like to be able to share with somebody, yes. I need a job to survive, but I don't need a man to survive."

"Yes, there are times when I think it would be really neat to meet somebody special that you can be with, go out and have a good time with," said Judy. "Once I thought I had to find somebody right away. But now I don't need to. There are times I feel a little romantic and I would like somebody there. Sometimes I'm a little frustrated. I did have the opportunity, he was serious, he wanted a commitment, but then he started making demands, moving in, 'This is how you do this.' I was showing my niece how to work a camera and he took the camera right out of my hands and started showing her himself. I said, 'Hey, back up, Charlie Brown, I've done this before and I don't want it.' "

Another dichotomy in sexy women appears over the issue of whether or not they use their sexual attractiveness to get advantages for themselves, or to get a man to do them a favor.

Some of the women who filled out my questionnaire refused to answer the section on using their sexual attractiveness. Many who did checked two opposite items—*"I never use my sexual attractiveness in this way,"* and also *"I use my attractiveness occsionally, in harmless ways."*

RuthAnn is in her 50s now, still an extremely attractive woman who has always drawn men, and who wears a humongous diamond on her right hand, a gift from a former lover. "I love to drive my car fast," she told me once. "I mean really *fast.* So I had to learn how to get out of traffic tickets, and here is how I do it. This works a whole lot better when you're alone. I just keep an atomizer of perfume in the console beside me, and when I'm pulled over, the first thing I do is reach for that atomizer and spray it in the air. Then I look up at the police officer and smile and bat my eyes at him. . . "

"I've never had a ticket in my life," said Sue, 36. "I don't do anything sexy, I just say 'yes, sir, no, sir,' but I use my eyes, I do turn on the charm. I was stopped in Rochester after three drinks, driving my son's car of all things, and when I was stopped and I wound the car window down, I told the officer, 'I'm so glad you stopped me. I'm in my son's car and I can't turn off the bright lights, can you show me how?' I asked him to show me twice so I could be sure I'd get it. . . . I thanked him and he let me go. If I'd had on curlers and no make-up and a hideous shirt, it wouldn't have worked nearly as well."

Thirteen of the women I surveyed admitted using their attractiveness to get out of a traffic citation, but the most common way they used their attractiveness ("I prefer to think of it as charm," one woman said) was to get a man to help them with a job or chore. "To get a man to take you someplace you wanted or needed to go," was the next most common way of using sexiness to wheedle something from a man.

Last October, when I was on a book tour, I saw another woman use her sex appeal very effectively to get a radio station to pay her some money. Caren was being paid by my publisher to drive me for the day, and she made a strategic error when she accidentally parked in a towaway zone. When we emerged from the radio station, her car was missing. She telephoned the towaway company and was told the bill would be $85, nearly the entire day's pay for Caren. She was upset, especially since she had parked in that lot on the instructions of the radio station itself.

Caren and I went back into the station, where she asked to speak to the manager. Two men came out to see what the problem was. Looking pretty, humble, and appealingly upset, Caren told her story, explaining that a secretary from the radio station had told her to park in that lot.

This was Atlanta, where chivalry still reigns, and the more upset Caren seemed, the more troubled both men looked. She had struck just the right note of feminine appeal. Finally she batted moist eyes at them and said in a soft voice, "So I don't know what to do. I guess I have to say, 'help.' What should I do?"

Effectively, she had thrown herself on their mercy, a plea I knew the two men were not going to be able to resist. Sure enough, after much going and coming and consulting, the results of Caren's appeals were that the radio station paid half of her towaway fee, and gave us a ride to the place where the car had been taken.

Afterwards, Caren admitted to being angry—she thought the radio station should have paid the whole towaway fee. Still, she also felt sheepishly proud of herself that she had managed to get any money at all. Single and a freelance publicist, Caren has had to survive on her wits, and she is not above using her sexiness in small ways, if it comes to that.

More than half of the women I quizzed said that they use their attractiveness "occasionally, in harmless ways." Eighteen women said that "men seem to enjoy it when I ask them little favors," and the same number said that "I don't see anything wrong with using my sexual appeal if it doesn't hurt anyone else."

Body Changes and Sex Appeal

The sense of her own sexiness in a woman is flexible, like a rubber net, and "bounces back" quickly after surgery that many consider catastrophic. Take mastectomies, for instance. One plastic surgeon told me that it takes most women *6 to 10 weeks* after breast surgery, whether or not they've had reconstruction, to gain back their body image, and incorporate the changes made in their body into their new pictures of themselves. In other words, to feel complete and womanly again.

One woman, Susan Jordan, wrote about her inspiring story. She was not only over 40, but she had had a double mastectomy and breast reconstruction. One day she took a look at herself in the mirror. What she saw was discouraging.

"Now, I had two beautiful breasts," Jordan wrote, "which looked like those of a twenty-year-old woman, so firm and upright that I would never have to wear a bra again. But the rest of my body was thin and shapeless and weak. I looked like a pencil with wonderful breasts!"

At that point, Jordan's new husband, Pat, suggested that she work out with weights. She could become a bodybuilder, and shape up her flabby arms and thighs.

Jordan visited a gym where "huge men stalked back and forth in front of mirrored walls, flexing chests, arms, thighs. Other men strained to lift iron bar bells. I heard screams of pain and harsh, clanging noises. . . . "

But Jordan didn't leave. Instead she stayed for what she later learned was a light workout—a session that left her unconditioned body gasping and sick to her stomach. She worked out for an hour and a half, four days a week. And received her reward several years later when she participated in a "Hot Bod" contest. The criteria was the body in the best shape, and Susan Jordan was a sensation. Shaking, nervous, she walked in her three-inch heels past an audience that was wildly cheering and blowing boat whistles for her.

The announcer paused, waiting for a little quiet. Then he said, "You will not believe this! This lady is forty-five years old!" At that point applause roared loose again. "Way to go!" shouted a woman of Jordan's own age.

The happy ending here is that Jordan had not only bested her age, but she had also turned surgery that many would consider "tragic" and "disfiguring" into a triumph.[26] And research has shown that this phenomenon is not only possible but *normal,* and is especially strong in women, who apparently have flexible senses of their own sexiness.

A loving partner can help inestimably in giving a woman back her own sense of body appeal. One woman writer told me about her "remarkable husband," who helped her get through her mastectomy with her spirit intact. "From Day One he joked with me that he was a butt man, not a breast man, and he meant it. He showed no distaste at my appearance, and the surgery made no difference in our sex life. We had a great romp the day I came home from the hospital."

Pregnancy is another event that also alters a woman's body image, even if only temporarily. However, pregnant women quickly learn to like their new, distended bodies. Jacqueline Fawcett, at the University of Pennsylvania School of Nursing, decided to test the age-old theory that pregnant women suffer from negative body images and hate their temporary bulges.

Fawcett studied a group of pregnant women ranging in age from 21 to 37. She found that in most cases the women had pretty accurate perceptions about their increasing girth, but the knowledge that they were getting bigger didn't seem to bother them. The researchers found no strongly negative attitudes— but, instead, acceptance.[27]

Another group of researchers studied patients who had os-tomy surgery, where a new excretory conduit is created in the abdomen. The individual is suddenly faced with a a massive psychological adjustment—he or she actually has a new body opening called a stoma. Forty-eight colostomy patients were extensively interviewed, and what they revealed was inspiring. Although 60 percent felt a decrease in their feelings of sexual attractiveness in the first year after surgery, in the year following, 67 percent gained most of those feelings back. Interestingly, it was the women who experienced the biggest regrowth in their feelings of sexiness, not the men.[28]

Aging is another body change that hits all women, causing mixed feelings and—finally—acceptance. "Our youth-loving culture discards fading beauty fast," says feminist Letty Cottin Pogrebin, "Especially fading females. For the woman accustomed to adulation and a greased track, it is a rude shock to be unseen or suddenly treated on the merits of performance rather than the accident of looks. And if the beauty never developed other strengths, what remains after the fading is a pitiful shell."[29]

Apparently, fewer and fewer aging women these days are allowing themselves to become "pitiful shells." Recently I appeared on the Oprah Winfrey show, which, that day, featured women over 40. The panel of 6 guests were all over 40, and so was the studio audience—in fact, the only ones under that age were Oprah herself, and some camera technicians. As the lively Oprah first quizzed her guests then roamed with a mike through the audience it became increasingly clear that every woman in that studio was happy with herself *as she was,* and *where she was in time.* Woman after woman raved about being 40, saying they felt the best they had ever felt in their lives. They felt sexy and alive and vital. It was an illuminating and uplifting experience.

Like many of the women I talked to, Cara, 41, told me a triumphant story of growth and happiness as the years progressed. "When I was married I was very disappointed in sex and felt frigid. I was married at 19, a virgin and all that. I used to read books on frigidity and came to the conclusion that I enjoyed closeness and touching, but that was all. After I became single, I had a beautiful, beautiful relationship and discovered that I'm not frigid at all. In fact, I am extremely multi-orgasmic. The difference is vast! I mean, when I was married, I was flat-chested. My ex used to make fun of me, used to tell me that I should sew up the front of my low-cut dress, I was the butt of many, many jokes. But after I got my divorce I underwent an actual physical change. I'm a C cup now. As soon as I got rid of him, I grew up—and I grew."

But as the population ages, the limits of sexiness are being pushed back even further than 40. Gloria Steinem recently wrote, "Fifty is what 40 used to be. The frontier of sexuality is being pushed back too. From Angie Dickinson to Cicely Tyson . . . women who already have passed or are about to reach 50 are remaining whole and sexual people in the public eye."[30]

I was even more touched to interview several dozen women from the Detroit Women Writers, a group of professional women writers. These are vibrant, "alive" women who, if single, never lack for male companions, and if widowed, often remarry no matter what their age. Many of them are in their 60s, some in their 70s, yet they had *all* come to a reasonably happy acceptance of themselves.

One woman, seventyish, has been attractive to men even recently. "My body?" she wrote. "Well, I'm glad I'm a size 8, after having been so much bigger for so long. Because of the ravages of time and of the surgical knife, I like my body better with clothes on. I comfort myself with the knowledge that I have good skin, and that my nails are beautifully shaped. I'm sorry my legs are gone. The thighs aren't bad, but knees and calves have sagged. I'm glad I have a short body and small ass, so the seat of slacks isn't halfway down to my knees, or bulging like oversized buns."

Another woman of 55 told me, "My daughter said recently while changing into her bathing suit and changing the baby into hers, 'I have to go get in the pool with Jeff's slender girlfriend.' 'Well, Renee,' I said while getting into my sturdy suit. 'I have to get into the pool with you.' I wanted her to know that while there's always someone younger and thinner, there's also someone older and plumper."

As these women demonstrate, aging can be accepted and incorporated into body image, and Raquel Welch perhaps epitomized the feelings of many women when she told *Paris Match* that she thought 42 was "a nice age."

"It is an age when one is no longer afraid. No longer afraid of other people's glances, no longer afraid of not always being thought the most beautiful person in the world. Obviously I hope I'm not a shrivelled old crone when I'm old, but I am far less afraid of growing old than I used to be. Do you know when I was nineteen I was terrified of the idea of being twenty-five. Today I have some white hairs, but I don't care. I don't dye them, in fact I think they are pretty. When you feel good, it is no longer so terrible to grow old. Personally, I feel like a rough diamond which has just been cut. I shine at last!"[31]

Axioms of Sex Appeal

1. Most of the sexy women I interviewed said they didn't feel they were doing anything special to be sexy.

2. Nearly all of the women said they would advise a daughter to achieve on her own merits and enjoy her own sex appeal, but the third most frequently marked statement was, "Be careful you don't allow men to use you."

3. Catcalls and whistles, annoyances sexy women regularly put up with, are viewed by some men as "flirting." If a woman wants

to avoid being catcalled, she should not smile, and should walk at a brisk, business-like pace.

4. Women with exceptional beauty are treated differently right from childhood. People assume that their beauty means they have other desirable personality characteristics. But beautiful women are targets for "beauty junkies" and harbor the fear that men may want them only for their looks.

5. On the other hand, plain women can take comfort in the fact that their love affairs may take longer to develop, and men are more likely to love them for themselves. The more average-looking woman should catalog her own personal beauty assets, and realize that sex appeal—according to men—doesn't necessarily correlate with beauty.

6. Sexy women carry a delicate balance between needing a man and being able to survive without one—which probably creates a sensuous unrest that men find appealing.

7. Many sexy women do use their "charm" or sexual attractiveness to get small advantages for themselves. Some don't want to admit this, and others believe that using their sexiness in small ways is harmless.

8. When a woman experiences major body changes caused by childbirth, surgery, etc., she is usually able to bounce back after a period of time into a renewed confidence in her own femininity.

9. Fewer and fewer women are finding aging a tragedy, and in fact, as the population grows older, the age limits of sexiness are being pushed back, to the point where 50 is what 40 once was. As Raquel Welch has said, "When you feel good, it is no longer so terrible to grow old. Personally, I feel like a rough diamond which has just been cut. I shine at last!"

Chapter Notes

Chapter 1

1. William Bolitho, *Camera Obscura,* New York, Simon & Schuster, 1930, p. 102.
2. Ellen Frank and Sandra Forsyth Enos, "Advice From America's Sexiest Wives," *Ladies Home Journal,* May 1983, pp. 62–126.
3. Martha Saxton, *Jayne Mansfield and the American Fifties,* Boston, Houghton Mifflin Co., 1975, p. 98.
4. Richard B. Sheridan, quoted in *2715 Quotations for Speakers, Writers and Raconteurs,* by Edward F. Murphy, New York, Crown Publishers, p. 22.
5. Anthony Summers, *Goddess: The Secret Lives of Marilyn Monroe,* New York, New American Library, 1986, p. 59.
6. *Ibid,* pp. 40–41.
7. Karen Stabiner, "Scintillating Cybill Shepherd," *McCalls,* March 1986, p. 105.
8. Richard David Story, "Meet Moviedom's Princess Kelly," *USA Weekend,* May 23–25, 1986, p. 4.
9. William Dunn, "U.S.A. Aging; New Median Age 31.8," *USA Today,* Wednesday, March 11, 1987, p. 1.
10. Joanne Austin, "What A Maturing Customer Means to Toiletries and Cosmetics Marketers," *Magazine Age,* July 1984, pp. 17–25.
11. *Ibid,* p. 25.
12. Wendy Leigh, *What Makes A Woman G.I.B. (Good In Bed),* New York, Penthouse Press, Ltd., 1977.

13. Brigitte Nioche, "What Men Want," *Penthouse,* July 1985, pp. 120–126.

Chapter 2

1. Janet L. Hopson, *Scent Signals: The Silent Language of Sex,* New York, William Morrow and Co., 1979, p. 98.
2. *Ibid,* p. 135.
3. *Ibid,* p. 139.
4. *Ibid,* p. 89.
5. James Hassett, "Sex and Smell," *Psychology Today,* March 1978, pp. 40–42.
6. Hopson, p. 141.
7. *Ibid,* p. 79.
8. Hassett, *op cit.* Also Hopson, pp. 127–129.
9. *Ibid.* Also Hopson, pp. 127–129.
10. Tom Robbins, *Even Cowgirls Get the Blues,* Boston, Houghton Mifflin, 1976, p. 351.
11. Peter Evans, *Bardot: Eternal Sex Goddess.* New York, Drake Publishers, Inc., 1973, p. 70.

Chapter 3

1. Lois W. Banner, *American Beauty,* New York, Knopf, 1983.
2. Francesco Scavullo, quote printed in *2715 One-Line Quotations for Speakers, Writers and Raconteurs,* by Edward F. Murphy, New York, Crown, p. 22.
3. Vincent Bozzi, "Choose Me," *Psychology Today,* August 1986, p. 66.
4. William A. Rossi, *The Sex Life of the Foot and Shoe,* New York, Saturday Review Press/E.P. Dutton, 1976, p. 173.
5. *Ibid,* p. 173.
6. Leigh, p. 65.
7. *Ibid,* p. 108.
8. *Ibid,* p. 46.
9. *Ibid,* p. 52.
10. *Ibid,* p. 59.

11. Rossi, p. 178.

12. H. J. Eysenck and Glenn Wilson, *The Psychology of Sex,* London, J. M. Dent & Sons, Ltd., 1979, p. 100.

13. Peg Bracken, *The Compleat I Hate To Cook Book,* Harcourt Brace Jovanovich, 1986.

14. Peter Manso, "Body Girls," *Penthouse,* June 1985, pp. 71–121.

15. Shari Miller Sims, "Diet Madness," *Vogue,* May 1986, p. 317.

16. Eysenck, pp. 49–50.

17. Quoted in *2715 One-Line Quotations for Speakers, Writers and Raconteurs,* by Edward F. Murphy, New York, Crown, p. 28.

18. Gary Stern, "Some Men Like Their Girlfriends Heavy, Dating Service Discovers," *Detroit News,* May 21, 1986, p. C-1.

19. Eysenck, p. 103.

20. Desmond Morris, *Body Watching,* New York, Crown Publishers, 1985.

21. Eysenck, p. 105.

22. Morris.

23. Lucy Freeman, *What Do Women Want? Self-Discovery Through Fantasy,* New York, Human Sciences Press, 1978, pp. 76–77.

24. Otis James, *Dolly Parton, A Personal Portrait,* New York, Quick Fox, 1978, p. 33.

25. Eysenck, pp. 50–51.

26. Anthony Leonard, "In Praise of Small Breasts," *Forum,* May 1983, pp. 27–37.

27. Eysenck, pp. 38–39.

28. Rossi, op cit.

Chapter 4

1. Frank, pp. 62–126.

2. Claire Rayner, "Sexual Chemistry," *New Woman,* May 1985, p. 63.

3. Leigh, p. 122.

4. Fred Robbins, "Joan Collins: I Feel Sorry For Men," *Redbook,* March 1986, p. 84.

5. Kathy Brown, "Even When I'm Thin I Feel Fat," *Mademoiselle,* April 1985, p. 229.

6. Frank, *op cit,* pp. 62–126.

7. Jacqueline Simenaur and David Carroll, "Sex and Singles; How Far Will They Go?" *Penthouse,* April 1982, p. 134.

8. Helen Andelin, *Fascinating Womanhood,* New York, Bantam Books, 1975, p. 67.

9. Summers, pp. 81–82.

10. Eysenck, p. 101.

11. Simenaur, p. 102.

12. Carol Austin Bridgewater, "Do Sexually Active Women Have Less Character?" *Psychology Today,* May 1983, p. 22.

13. Frank, *op cit,* pp. 62–126.

14. Letty Cottin Pogrebin, "The Power of Beauty: A Feminist Wrestles With the Indisputable "Fact" That Looks Do Count," *Ms.,* December 1983, p. 75.

Chapter 5

1. Stabiner, *op cit,* p. 105.

2. Rossi, p. 141.

3. *Ibid,* p. 138.

4. Laura Fissinger, *Tina Turner,* New York, Ballantine, 1985, pp. 96–97.

5. Julius Fast, *Body Language,* New York, M. Evans Co., 1970, p. 45–63.

6. *Ibid,* pp. 45–63.

7. Adrienne Munich, "Seduction in Academe," *Psychology Today,* February 1978, pp. 82–84.

8. Gerald L. Clore, *et al.,* "Judging Attraction from Nonverbal Behavior: The Gain Phenomenon," *Journal of Consulting and Clinical Psychology,* 1975, vol. 43, No. 4, pp. 491–497.

9. Constance Backhouse and Leah Cohen, *Sexual Harassment on the Job,* Englewood Cliffs, N.J., Prentice-Hall, Inc., 1981, pp. 158–161.

10. David B. Givens, "The Nonverbal Basis of Attraction: Flirtation, Courtship and Seduction," *Psychiatry,* vol. 41, November 1978, pp. 346–359.

11. Charles Bowney, "Flirting—Some Quick Ways to Break the Ice," *Detroit News,* April 4, 1986, p. C-1.

12. Paul McCarthy, "First Moves," *Psychology Today*, October 1986, p. 12.

Chapter 6

1. Givens, *op cit*, pp. 346–359.
2. *Ibid*, pp. 346–359.
3. *Ibid*, pp. 346–359.
4. *Ibid*, pp. 346–359.
5. Hans Hass, *The Human Animal: The Mystery of Man's Behavior*, New York, G. P. Putnam's Sons, 1970.
6. Morris.
7. George Eels and Stanley Musgrove, *Mae West: A Biography*, New York, William Morrow & Co., 1982, p. 126.
8. Julius Fast and Meredith Bernstein, *Sexual Chemistry: What It Is, How to Use It*, New York, M. Evans Co., 1983, p. 29.
9. Fast, *Body Language*, pp. 33–37.
10. Charles Downey, "Flirting—Some Quick Ways to Break the Ice," *Detroit News*, April 4, 1986, p. C-1.
11. Linda Lee and James Charlton, "The Not-So-Subtle Art of Seduction," *New Woman*, October 1984, pp. 84–87.
12. Desmond Morris, "Sexy Hair Gestures," *Self*, September 1985, pp. 170–171.
13. Givens, *op cit*, pp. 346–359.

Chapter 7

1. Lorna J. Sarrell and Philip M. Sarrell, *Sexual Turning Points: the Seven Stages of Adult Sexuality*, New York, Macmillan, 1984, pp 14–16.
2. Susan Brownmiller, *Femininity*, New York, Simon & Schuster, 1984, p. 41.
3. Elaine Walster, et al., "Playing Hard To Get: Understanding an Elusive Phenomenon," *Journal of Personality and Social Psychology*, 1973, vol. 26, No. 1, pp. 113–121.
4. *Ibid*, pp. 113–121.
5. Clore, *op cit*, p. 491–497.

6. Donald G. Dutton and Arthur P. Aron, "Some Evidence for Heightened Sexual Attraction Under Conditions of High Anxiety," *Journal of Personality and Social Psychology,,* 1974, vol. 30, No. 4, pp. 510–517.

7. *Ibid,* pp. 510–517.

8. *Ibid,* pp. 510–517.

9. Eysenck, p. 124.

10. Nancy C. Baker, "The Beauty Trap," *New Woman,* April 1985, pp. 74–76.

11. James W. Pennebaker, "Truckin' With Country-Western Psychology," *Psychology Today,* November 1979, p. 18.

12. Frank Beach, "It's All In Your Mind," *Psychology Today,* July 1969, p. 88.

13. Vincent Bozzi, "Beauty By Association," *Psychology Today,* September 1985, p. 66.

Chapter 8

1. Frank, *op cit,* pp. 62–126.

2. Carol Tavris and Susan Sadd, *The Redbook Report on Female Sexuality,* New York, Delacorte Press, 1975, pp. 218–233.

3. Robert Athanasiou, et al., "Sex," *Psychology Today,* July 1970, p. 87.

4. Eysenck, pp. 168–171.

5. *Ibid,* pp. 168.

6. *Ibid,* pp. 168.

7. Joyce Brothers, *What Every Woman Should Know About Men,* New York, Simon & Schuster, 1981, p. 156.

8. Tavris, pp. 218–233.

9. Frank, *op cit,* p. 62–126.

10. *Ibid,* p. 62–126.

11. Tavris, *op cit,* pp. 218–233.

12. Leigh, p. 118.

13. Leigh, p. 79.

14. Ken Druck, "Secrets Men Keep About Sex," *Family Circle,* October 15, 1985, p. 40.

15. Nioche, *op cit,* p. 120–126.

16. Frank, *op cit*, p. 62–126.
17. E. Barbara Hariton, "The Sexual Fantasies of Women," *Psychology Today*, March 1973, p. 52.
18. *Ibid*, p. 52.
19. Kathryn Falk, *How To Write A Romance And Get It Published*, New York, Crown Publishers, 1983, p. 113.
20. Vincent Bozzi, "Sex And The Romance Reader," *Psychology Today*, November 1985, p. 73.

Chapter 9

1. Saxton, *op cit*, pp. 98–118.
2. Carolyn See, "Hers," *New York Times*, July 10, 1986, p. 14.
3. Andelin, pp. 155–157.
4. Eysenck, p. 101.
5. Leigh, p. 74.
6. *Upon Julia's Clothes*, by Robert Herrick, reprinted in *Viking Book of Poetry of the English Speaking World*, Richard Aldington Ed., Viking Press, New York, p. 328.
7. Priscilla Beaulieu Presley, "Elvis and Me," *Ladies Home Journal*, October 1985, p. 62.
8. Ray Fullaga, "What Your Favorite Color Reveals About You," *New Woman*, March 1985, p. 156.
9. Rossi, p. 90.
10. *Ibid*, p. 120.
11. Brownmiller, p. 186.
12. Rossi, p. 91.
13. *Ibid*, p. 91–100.
14. Linda Stasi, *Looking Good Is the Best Revenge,*, New York, St. Martin's/Marek, 1984, pp. 60–61.
15. *Delight in Disorder*, by Robert Herrick, reprinted in *Viking Book of Poetry of the English Speaking World*, Richard Aldington, Ed., Viking Press, New York, p. 325.
16. Manso, *op cit*, pp. 71–121.
17. "The Hair Men Love Most," *Woman's Day*, October 21, 1986, p. 39.

18. "Make-up Makes You More Memorable," *Self,* March, 1985, p. 40.

19. Frank, *op cit,* pp. 62–126.

Chapter 10

No footnotes

Chapter 11

1. Peter Evans, *Bardot: Eternal Sex Goddess,* New York, Drake Publishers, Inc., 1973, pp. 130–131.

2. Frank, *op cit,* pp. 62–126.

3. Baker, *op cit,* pp. 74–76.

4. *Ibid,* pp. 74.

5. *Ibid,* pp. 74–76.

6. Robert Karen, "Sex and Work," *Cosmopolitan,* July 1986, pp. 186–189.

7. Nioche, *op cit,* pp. 120–126.

8. Backhouse, p. 117.

9. Liz Roman Gallese, *Women Like Us: What Is Happening to the Women of the Harvard Business School Class of '75—The Women Who Had the First Chance to Make It to the Top,* New York, William Morrow and Co., 1985.

10. Irene Pickhardt, "Oh, You Beautiful Doll!" *Parents,,* October 1983, pp. 72–74.

11. Carol Pogash, "Real Live Dolls: When Pretty Babies Play the Beauty Pageant Game," *Redbook,* June 1984, pp. 91–93.

12. Stabiner, *op cit,* p. 105.

13. Pogrebin, pp. 75–109.

14. Michael Korda, *Worldly Goods,* New York, Random House, 1982, p. 81.

15. Ross Wetzsteon, "Men Who Are Hooked On Looks," *Mademoiselle,,* August 1983, pp. 190–289.

16. Peter Haining, *Raquel Welch: Sex Symbol to Superstar,* New York, St. Martin's Press, 1984, p. 35.

17. *Ibid,* p. 133.

18. *Ibid,* p. 179.

19. Summers, p. 415.

20. Saxton, p. 119.

21. *Ibid,* p. 99.

22. James, p. 33.

23. Ellen Seton, "What's So Great About Being Average Looking? Plenty!" *Mademoiselle,,* February 1984, p. 188.

24. Saxton, p. 99.

25. Evans, p. 75.

26. Susan Ryan Jordan, "Overcoming My Mastectomy with Body-building," *Cosmopolitan,* November 1985, p. 224.

27. Jacqueline Fawcett, "Pretty Big," *Health,* June 1986, p. 6.

28. Nancy Fugate Woods, *Human Sexuality in Health and Illness,* St. Louis, The C. V. Mosby Company, 1979, pp. 193–335.

29. Pogrebin, pp. 75–109.

30. Jane O'Reilly, "A Candle at 50, For Accomplishment," *New York Times,* July 10, 1986, p. C-10.

31. Haining, p. 168.

Bibliography

Andelin, Helen B. *Fascinating Womanhood.* New York: Bantam Books, 1975.

Athanasiou, Robert, et al. "Sex: (response to P.T. Questionnaire)", *Psychology Today,* July 1970.

Austin, Joanne. "What A Maturing Consumer Means to Toiletries and Cosmetics Marketers," *Magazine Age,* July 1984.

Bach, George R., and Deutsch, Ronald M. *Pairing: How to Achieve Genuine Intimacy.* New York: Peter H. Wyden, Inc., 1970.

Backhouse, Constance, and Cohen, Leah. *Sexual Harassment on the Job.* Englewood Cliffs, N.J.: Prentice-Hall, Inc., 1981.

Baker, Nancy C. "The Beauty Trap," *New Woman,* April 1985.

Banner, Lois W. *American Beauty.* New York: Knopf, 1983.

Beach, Frank. "It's All In Your Mind," *Psychology Today,* July 1969.

Berne, Eric. *Sex In Human Loving.* New York: Simon & Schuster, 1970.

Berscheid, Ellen, and Walster, Elaine. "Beauty and the Beast," *Psychology Today,* March 1972.

Berscheid, Ellen, et al. "Physical Attractiveness and Dating Choice: A Test of the Matching Hypothesis," *Journal of Experimental Social Psychology,* 1971, vol. 7, pp. 173–189.

Blotnik, Srully. *Otherwise Engaged: The Private Lives of Successful Career Women.* New York: Facts on File Publications, 1985.

Bozzi, Vincent. "Beauty by Association," *Psychology Today,* August 1985.

Bozzi, Vincent. "Body Talk," *Psychology Today,* September 1985.

Bozzi, Vincent. "Sex and the Romance Reader," *Psychology Today,* November 1985.

Bridgewater, Carol Austin. "Do Sexually Active Women Have Less Character?" *Psychology Today,* May 1983.

Brothers, Joyce. *What Every Woman Should Know About Men.* New York: Simon & Schuster, 1981.

Brown, Kathy. "Even When I'm Thin I Feel Fat," *Mademoiselle,* April 1985.

Brownmiller, Susan. *Femininity.* New York: Simon & Schuster, 1984.

Burns, David D. *Intimate Connections,* New York: William Morrow & Co., 1985.

Cash, Thomas F. and Janda, Louis H. "The Eye of the Beholder," *Psychology Today,* December 1984.

Clore, Gerald L., et al. "Judging Attraction from Nonverbal Behavior: The Gain Phenomenon," *Journal of Consulting and Clinical Psychology,* 1975, vol. 43, No. 4.

———. "What Men Think . . . The Gallup Organization Surveyed Hundreds of Single Men on the Subject of Women . . . And This Is What They Found!" *Cosmopolitan,* November 1985.

Dermer, Marshall and Thiel, Darrel L. "When Beauty May Fail," *Journal of Personality and Social Psychology,* 1975, vol. 31, No. 6.

Dion, Karen, et al. "What Is Beautiful Is Good," *Journal of Personality and Social Psychology,* 1972, vol. 24, No. 3.

Druck, Ken. "Secrets Men Keep About Sex," *Family Circle,* October 15, 1985.

Dutton, Donald G., and Aron, Arthur P. "Some Evidence For Heightened Sexual Attraction Under Conditions of High Anxiety," *Journal of Personality and Social Psychology,* 1974, vol. 30, No. 4.

Eels, George and Musgrove, Stanley. *Mae West: A Biography.* New York: William Morrow & Co., 1982.

Evans, Peter. *Bardot: Eternal Sex Goddess.* New York: Drake Publishers Inc., 1973.

Eysenck, H. J. and Wilson, Glenn. *The Psychology of Sex.* London: J. M. Dent & Sons, Ltd., 1979.

Falk, Kathryn. *How To Write A Romance And Get It Published,* New York: Crown Publishers, 1983.

Fast, Julius. *Body Language*. New York: M. Evans Co., 1970.

Fast, Julius, and Bernstein, Meredith. *Sexual Chemistry: What It Is, How To Use It*. New York: M. Evans Co., 1983.

Fawcett, Jacqueline. "Pretty Big," *Health*, June 1986.

Fischer, Arlene. "Who Ages Well—And Why," *Redbook*, May 1986.

Fissinge, Laura. *Tina Turner*. New York: Ballantine, 1985.

Frank, Ellen, and Enos, Sandra Forsyth. "Advice From America's Sexiest Wives," *Ladies Home Journal*, May 1983.

Freeman, Lucy. *What Do Women Want? Self-Discovery Through Fantasy*. New York: Human Sciences Press, 1978.

Fullaga, Ray. "What Your Favorite Color Reveals About You," *New Woman*, March 1985.

Gallese, Liz Roman. *Women Like Us: What Is Happening to the Women of the Harvard Business School Class of '75—The Women Who Had the First Chance to Make It to the Top*. New York: William Morrow and Co., 1985.

Gallucci, Nicholas T., and Meyer, Robert G. "People Can Be Too Perfect: Effects of Subjects' and Targets' Attractiveness on Interpersonal Attraction," *Psychological Reports*, 1984, vol. 55.

Givens, David B. "The Nonverbal Basis of Attraction: Flirtation, Courtship and Seduction," *Psychiatry*, vol. 41, November, 1978.

Gloeckner, Mary Reid. "Perceptions of Sexual Attractiveness Following Ostomy Surgery," *Research in Nursing and Health*, 1984, vol. 7.

Haining, Peter. *Raquel Welch: Sex Symbol to Superstar*. New York: St. Martin's Press, 1984.

Hariton, E. Barbara. "The Sexual Fantasies of Women," *Psychology Today*, March 1973.

Hartman, Rose. *Birds of Paradise: An Intimate View of the New York Fashion World*. New York: Dell Publishing, 1980.

Hass, Hans. *The Human Animal: The Mystery of Man's Behavior*. New York: G. P. Putnam's Sons, 1970.

Hassett, James. "Sex and Smell," *Psychology Today*, March 1978.

Heiman, Julia R. "Women's Sexual Arousal: The Physiology of Erotica," *Psychology Today*, April 1975.

Hopson, Janet L. *Scent Signals: The Silent Language of Sex*. New York: William Morrow and Co., 1979.

James, Otis. *Dolly Parton, A Personal Portrait*. New York: Quick Fox, 1978.

Johnson, Catherine. "Physical Attraction: How Much Do His Looks Affect Your Feelings—and Vice Versa?" *Self*, August 1985.

Jordan, Susan Ryan. "Overcoming My Mastectomy With Bodybuilding," *Cosmopolitan*, November 1985.

Kahn, Elayne J. and Rudnitsky, David A. *1001 Ways You Reveal Your Personality*, New York: New American Library, 1982.

Kaplan, Helen Singer. "Do Other Women Enjoy Sex More?" *Redbook*, April 1986.

Karen, Robert. "Sex And Work," *Cosmopolitan*, July 1986.

Lee, Linda, and Charlton, James. "The Not-So-Subtle Art of Seduction," *New Woman*, October 1984.

Leigh, Wendy. *What Makes A Woman G.I.B. (Good In Bed)*. New York: Penthouse Press, Ltd., 1977.

Leonard, Anthony. "In Praise of Small Breasts," *Forum*, May 1983.

Levine-Schneideman, Conalee, and Levine, Karen. "Love Strategies: If We're So Smart, Why Aren't We Happy?" *Working Woman*, April 1985.

Liebowitz, Michael R. *The Chemistry of Love*. Boston: Little, Brown & Co., 1983.

Manso, Peter. "Body Girls," *Penthouse*, June 1985.

Marchant-Haycox, Susan. "What Your Walk Says About You," *New Woman*, May 1985.

McCarthy, Paul. "First Moves," *Psychology Today*, October 1986.

Mills, Bart. *Tina*. New York: Warner Books, 1985.

Morris, Desmond. *Body Watching*. New York: Crown Publishers, 1985.

Morris, Desmond. "Sexy Hair Gestures," *Self*, September 1985.

Munich, Adrienne. "Seduction in Academe," *Psychology Today*, February 1978.

Nioche, Brigitte. "What Men Want," *Penthouse*, July 1985.

Norwood, Robin. *Women Who Love Too Much: When You Keep Wishing And Hoping He'll Change*. New York: Jeremy P. Tarcher, Inc., 1985.

Pennebaker, James W. "Truckin' with Country-Western Psychology," *Psychology Today*, November 1979.

Pickhardt, Irene. "Oh, You Beautiful Doll!" *Parents*, October 1983.

Pogash, Carol. "Real Live Dolls: When Pretty Babies Play the Beauty Pageant Game," *Redbook*, June 1984.

Pogrebin, Letty Cottin. "The Power of Beauty: A Feminist Wrestles with the Indisputable "Fact" That Looks Do Count," *Ms.,* December 1983.

Presley, Priscilla Beaulieu. "Elvis and Me," *Ladies Home Journal,* October 1985.

Rayner, Claire. "Sexual Chemistry," *New Woman,* May 1985.

Robbins, Harold. *The Carpetbaggers.* New York: Pocket Books, 1961.

Rossi, William A. *The Sex Life of the Foot and Shoe.* New York: Saturday Review Press/E. P. Dutton, 1976.

Rubenstein, Carol. "Sex Repel," *Psychology Today,* December 1979.

Sarrell, Lorna J., and Sarrell, Philip M. *Sexual Turning Points: The Seven Stages of Adult Sexuality.* New York: Macmillan, 1984.

Saxton, Martha. *Jayne Mansfield and the American Fifties.* Boston: Houghton Mifflin Co., 1975.

Seton, Ellen. "What's So Great About Being Average Looking? Plenty!" *Mademoiselle,* February 1984.

Simenauer, Jacqueline, and Carroll, David. "Sex And Singles: How Far Will They Go?" *Penthouse,* April 1982.

Sims, Shari Miller. "Diet Madness," *Vogue,* May 1986.

Stasi, Linda. *Looking Good is the Best Revenge.* New York: St. Martin's/Marek, 1984.

Summers, Anthony. *Goddess: The Secret Lives of Marilyn Monroe.* New York: Macmillan, 1985.

Tannahill, Reay. *Sex in History.* New York: Stein and Day, 1980.

Tavris, Carol, and Sadd, Susan. *The Redbook Report on Female Sexuality.* New York: Delacorte Press, 1975.

Wallace, Irving, et al. *The Intimate Sex Lives of Famous People,* New York: Dell, 1982.

Walster, et al. "Playing Hard To Get: Understanding and Elusive Phemomenon," *Journal of Personality and Social Psychology,* 1973, vol. 26, No. 1.

Weaver, James B., et al. "Effect of Erotica on Young Men's Aesthetic Perception of their Female Sexual Partners," *Perceptual and Motor Skills,* 1984, vol. 58.

Wetzsteon, Ross. "Men Who Are Hooked On Looks," *Mademoiselle,* August, 1983.

"When Love and Sex Intrude at Work, Executives May Find It Harder to Get Down to Business," *People,* March 24, 1986.

Williams, Juanita H. *Psychology of Women: Behavior in a Biosocial Context.* New York: W. W. Norton and Co., Inc., 1974, 1977.

Woods, Nancy Fugate. *Human Sexuality in Health and Illness.* St. Louis: The C. V. Mosby Company, 1979.

Index